I Married A JUNKIE

The Final Chapter...
Til Death Do Us Part

DR. CALI ESTES
&
TIM ESTES
1/29/1970 - 1/9/2023

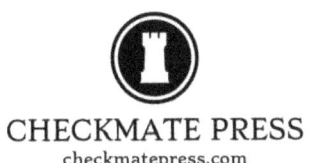

CHECKMATE PRESS
checkmatepress.com

Copyright © 2024 by **Dr. Cali Estes & Tim Estes**

All rights reserved. No part of this publication may be reproduced, distributed or transmitted in any form or by any means, without prior written permission.

Checkmate Press books are published by:

**McLean Media Group, LLC
101 Chestnut Grove Ave #7
Bozeman, MT 59718**

I Married A Junkie: The Final Chapter... Til Death Do Us Part / Dr. Cali Estes & Tim Estes. -- 1st ed.
ISBN 978-1-7321781-8-2

The Publisher has strived to be as accurate and complete as possible in the creation of this book.

This book is not intended for use as a source of legal, business, health, or medical advice. All readers are advised to seek services of competent professionals in legal, business, and health or medical fields.

While all attempts have been made to verify information provided in this publication, the Publisher assumes no responsibility for errors, omissions, or contrary interpretation of the subject matter herein. Any perceived slights of specific persons, peoples, or organizations are unintentional.

I Married A Junkie – The Final Chapter

This book is dedicated to every spouse of an active drug/alcohol user that is going through hell trying to get their loved one sober.

Dr. Cali Estes & Tim Estes

I Married A Junkie – The Final Chapter

CONTENTS

FOREWORD by Mike Tramp

INTRODUCTION   1

THE STORY   3

ACKNOWLEDGEMENTS   139

EPILOGUE   141

TALES FROM THE ROAD   145

THANK YOU   167

Dr. Cali Estes & Tim Estes

I Married A Junkie – The Final Chapter

Foreword

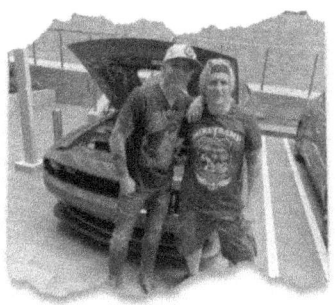

Everybody knows a Junkie.

It could be your best friend, your neighbor or someone hanging out in the street. For me it was my late brother, and it stayed with him throughout his 61 years. He was a sixties child and grew up as the neighborhood guinea pig. At 13 years old, he made his own tattoo in school with a razor blade and ink from a pen, and after that there was no stopping.

Copenhagen, Denmark was at the frontline of liberty and freedom, and the first country to legalize pornography, the first country in the world that made a sex change operation. My brother was right at home with no borders.

I wasn't aware when he started doing the hard drugs, and needles became a part of it, though he always somehow seemed to dodge the bullet. He managed to have big breaks from the addiction, and it would stay with him till his death. With the Danish government deciding to subsidize the local junkies with free methadone and fixing rooms where they could inject in peace and away from people to see it, why would anyone try to get clean?

Looking back at all of this, and at the same time I have now been in the Rock'n'Roll world for 46 years and seen it all. I wonder why it was my brother who took the wrong path and not me. I sure had it in front of me daily but was never tempted.

In the last years of his life, I would visit my mom, and my brother was there. Suddenly, in the middle of what we were doing or watching, he would go to the bathroom and disappear.

My mom would start getting nervous. When I witnessed it the first time, I ended up breaking down the bathroom door, only to find my brother on the floor with a needle in his arms. Then I started looking at it in a different way. If he could do this right in front of the ones who loved him, the need for a fix was way stronger than the pain and suffering he caused his mom. At that moment nothing else mattered to him but peace.

I once toured with one of the biggest rock stars in the world. He had lived that kind of life but got clean and was now on the right path. He said to me, "Mike it's not that I can't enjoy a beer with you or a glass of wine, but once it hits me, I want it all and I am going to go for it, without stopping. For the rest of my life that's how it's going to be, there is no letting down my guard."

Mike Tramp - Solo artist and original vocalist of White Lion and Freak of Nature

I Married A Junkie – The Final Chapter

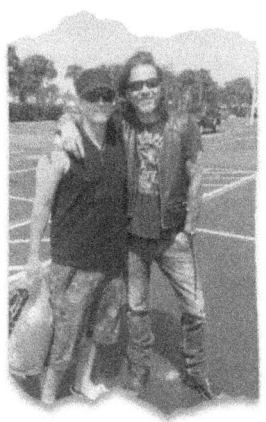

Suggested Listen: Need

Innocent soul, troubled mind
The needle pricks the skin
Close my eyes and fade away
Soon I'm in your world
It's peaceful here, just you and I
No one to fight or fear
Nothing matters, only me
My pain has disappeared

Only in your world can I dream
Escape from reality
The pain buried within
Only from your hands will I take
The love and life you offer me

Dr. Cali Estes & Tim Estes

The addiction I begin

Suddenly but quietly
You came upon me
A wolf in sheep's clothing
I let you close to me
And in disguise you told me lies
The friend I never had
I was weak, I gave up hope,
I desperately needed you

Only in your world can I dream......

My family and friends
I have caused a lot of pain
Their accusations I deny
But in my face they see my lies
Now I hang around your door
'Cause everyday I need you more
I need you more
I need you more

Only in your world can I dream......

Words and Music: Mike Tramp
From the Freak of Nature album "Gathering of Freaks"

Introduction

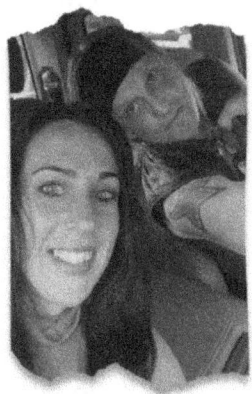

Welcome to *"I Married a Junkie: Book Two, The Final Chapter."*

Most books you read about addiction focus on parents dealing with an addicted child or coping with the loss of a child to overdose. Support groups often cater to parents of active addicts or those grieving a child lost to drug poisoning. Even grief groups do not focus on the loss of a spouse due to drug addiction or long-term use.

This book, however, is dedicated to the spouses of addicts – a group that is often overlooked and for whom few resources are available.

Many people believe that a spouse can simply walk away from an addict, file for divorce, and leave the situation, unlike a parent who can never truly leave their child. I'm going to debunk this theory.

It's not as easy to walk away from someone who descends into active addiction when you met them sober, shared several good years with, and came to know as your person. When they descend into the depths of drug addiction, you want your person back. Sometimes at any cost, even to your own health and wellbeing.

This book is dedicated to all the spouses of addicts who didn't leave, who did leave, or who watched their loved ones spiral out of control into addiction, possibly overdosing or dying from complications. What sets this story apart is that my husband, Tim Estes, didn't die from an overdose. He died from a heart attack after 29 days clean from fentanyl, due to long-term complications of drug use, including prolonged microdosing of fentanyl and crack cocaine (speedball use).

I hope this book will not only entertain you and remind you of Tim (he was writing the chapters when he passed), but also shed light on the living hell experienced by the partners of addicts. It aims to explore ways we can support these partners when their loved ones don't want to get clean.

After each chapter you will have the pleasure of listening to a song, the lyrics match the chapter. Plug it into your iTunes or Spotify and give it a listen.

As always, you can reach out to me, Dr. Cali Estes, at SoberOnDemand.com or call us at 1-800-706-0318 for help for yourself or a loved one suffering from addiction.

1
Tim

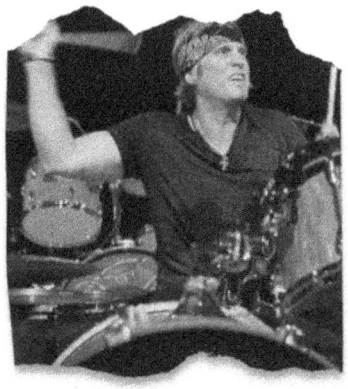

Imagine this, especially those of you who know anything about precipitated withdrawal. My beautiful wife loves the state of Alaska, and since our first trip up there went so well (which was graphically described in the first book), we decided to go again. This time it wasn't a summer trip - we were going in the fall.

Now, fall in Alaska for a Florida boy is not a pretty sight. I made the brilliant decision to take a few bags of heroin with me to "warm me up" while there. For me, a few bags mean about 30-40 nickel bags. Now, I was pretty good at math in school, and a true addict can run numbers like a certified accountant, especially when it comes to our daily intake of our favorite drug.

So, back to Liberty City I went to stock up for my big trip! This is the moment it all went south as I set myself up for a horrible experience. I scored my 40 nickel bags, and of course, I had to do three right then and there. What did you think - that I was going to wait until Alaska to get high? Not in a million years! I figured three wouldn't hurt me, as I still had 37 bags left. We were leaving the next day for Alaska with a short stop in Seattle for a Cowboys vs. Seahawks football game. Then it hit me - I forgot to factor in Seattle.

Here's what I planned to do: I still had a few Suboxone strips from when I last got clean. Suboxone stops withdrawal and binds to the opiate receptors in the brain to stop cravings. Blocking those receptors is the last thing I wanted to do. But I thought if I timed it right and didn't use anymore heroin until after Seattle, I could jump on Suboxone for just a dose or two.

That way, I wouldn't get sick or block my receptors, could enjoy the game, then stop the Suboxone. By the time we got to the airport in Seattle, I could jump back to heroin and be right on track. I convinced myself it was a perfect, flawless plan. I had to be the smartest guy I knew!

This Alaska trip was very important because I had royally messed up our first visit. I couldn't let my wife down again.

As I walked into our Miami condo, she asked how rehearsal went. Thank God she didn't suspect I had been out scoring dope for the trip - it would have been the end of me. She's Italian, from the Philly area. You do not want to piss off a female Italian from Philly, trust me on that one! Happy wife, happy high. I nodded off thinking my plan was foolproof.

At 4am, my eyes popped open. Our flight wasn't until 9am, and the airport was only 10 minutes away. I would have done anything for three more bags - early morning was always my favorite time to use. My wife was sound asleep, the bathroom just five feet from our bed. I told myself three more bags wouldn't throw off my plan. I had this under control...

Fifteen minutes later, I was down to 34 bags, and we hadn't even left the condo. Could I screw this up again? No way, I tried to convince myself. It was only 4:15am - plenty of time. And 34 bags were more than enough for a 5-day trip.

I just needed to relax, nod back off, and not stress.

The next thing I knew, my wife was shaking me violently, yelling at me to get up and shower because we were running late. What an unpleasant jolt that was. Keep the word "unpleasant" in mind as you read on because things quickly go from bad to worse.

A lot of crazy thoughts run through my head when using heroin. One recurring notion was that my wife always knew when I was high and would purposely put me in uncomfortable situations to ruin my high, make my withdrawal worse, and force me to quit for good. Could she really be that smart?

Maybe, but I was way smarter, I assured myself.

Like a good boy, I rolled out of bed and got in the shower. But wait - my favorite time to use is right before a hot shower. If I did three more bags, I'd still have 31 left for this short trip, which was plenty.

With the time change going west, I still had almost 24 hours before I'd need Suboxone. Nine bags in, my plan was still intact. I wouldn't get sick. I had this.

Three bags later, I was enjoying an amazing shower, lost in a beautiful nod as the hot water ran over me. Suddenly, another unpleasant jolt - my wife pounding on the door, yelling at me to get out and get dressed because the Uber would be there in 15 minutes.

That was twice now with the unpleasant interruptions. Did she know? No way, I convinced myself I was just being paranoid.

There we were - the Uber on the way, and I had 31 bags for my 5-day trip. I ran the numbers in my head - a little over seven bags a day. Remember, I wasn't using any more until Alaska, thanks to my brilliant Suboxone plan. I'd hit Anchorage with 31 bags, which was plenty for four days there.

I was right as rain, except for one thing - I hate odd numbers, and the Miami airport is my favorite place to use. Now I was in a bit of a pickle. One bag was a waste of time, but it would put me at an even 30 bags, my absolute cutoff for Alaska.

Then again, so would 28, and I always do three at a time... Three more it was, leaving me exactly seven per day for Alaska. I harmlessly eliminated that pesky fraction - not that it mattered in my world anyway. I was still good.

I Married A Junkie – The Final Chapter

We boarded our first-class seats. My wife always books us up front for better service, quicker loading/unloading, and comfort.

Not bad - I managed to get on the plane with 28 bags for my four days in Alaska. Except airplane bathrooms are my favorite place to use. There's something exhilarating about nodding at 33,000 feet - that's why they're my favorite!

I had no conscious thought that I had gone from 40 bags down to 25 before even leaving Miami. Active addiction has a funny way of tuning out those realizations.

The next thing I remember is the flight attendant waking me to put my seat up as we landed in Phoenix. I had completely forgotten about our 2-hour layover there, and Phoenix is another favorite place of mine to use.

Could I make 22 bags last through Alaska? Of course - not only was I the smartest guy I knew, but I was also a highly functioning addict. Three bags later in the Phoenix airport bathroom, I was feeling great!

Two hours after that, we were back at 33,000 feet, Seattle-bound. Ten minutes later, I was in the plane bathroom doing three more bags.

That's when the first twinges of worry crept in. Staring out the window, I realized I was in the danger zone with only 19 bags left, having done 21 since scoring the day before.

I was badly fucking up my brilliant plan. What I should have been focused on was how I was fucking up the trip and letting my wife down again, but no - I was only concerned about my crumbling plan.

I just needed to alter it slightly, I told myself. That's what I do on heroin - make necessary minor adjustments. To me they're minor; to a sane person they're life-threatening.

Okay, I tried to calm myself down. I was almost to Seattle, still had 19 bags, felt fine, and wasn't sick. I was only a day and a half from Alaska, and it seemed no one was onto me.

Remember when I mentioned the crazy thoughts heroin induces? Well, one split-second notion raced through my head, and a split-second was all my addicted mind needed to screw me over completely. I convinced myself to relax, that it was no big deal if I ran low on dope. I was headed to Seattle, the heroin capital of the U.S.!

I think I mentioned my Denver experience in the first book - I had run out of heroin there once, surprise surprise. I was hellbent on not going into withdrawal, even though I had never copped in Denver and didn't know anyone.

But I knew what to do - Google it! I literally searched "Where to buy heroin in Denver" and it told me to go to the Cherry Creek bike path downtown, look for South American guys flashing tiny balloons in their mouths, and flash my money. Did it work? You bet. Why not try the same in Seattle if needed?

Here was my minor adjustment: Thanks to my phone, I now knew I'd have to walk through a known drug area in Seattle to get from our hotel to the Seahawks stadium.

I figured I'd scope out the dope dealers on the way to the game but couldn't score then because my wife would be with me.

After the game, once we were back at the hotel, I'd offer to go grab us food. I'd run the 10 blocks to the drug zone, cop, run the 10 blocks back to the deli, grab the food, and be back on track.

Except Seattle is nothing like Denver. If they don't know you, the dealers won't give you the time of day. My phone had lied to me this time.

I failed miserably at scoring but still had to book it back to the deli. I grabbed our food and headed up to the room. I guess it wasn't as dire as it seemed - I still had 19 bags left, we were flying to Alaska the next day, and we were staying at a great hotel.

Then again, hotel rooms are my favorite place to use...

The next morning, I woke up to get ready for our Alaska flight with 16 bags to my name. I got in the shower - thirteen bags left. Called the Uber - ten bags. Back to the Seattle airport - seven bags. In our first-class seats - four bags left as I was self-destructing at warp speed. Then the airplane bathroom - one measly bag remaining. Screw it, one bag wouldn't fend off withdrawal, I did all four.

I returned to my seat with zero bags, still hours from Anchorage. I didn't need a minor adjustment - I needed a fucking miracle!

Panic set in hard. What started as a brilliant, foolproof plan had devolved into snorting 40 bags in just over 48 hours. Now I was hurtling at 500mph in the opposite direction of Miami, about to be the furthest I could possibly be from it within the U.S. There I was, in my usual fucked up spot, the entire Alaska trip about to implode.

My wife was sound asleep, first class was packed, it was pitch black outside with a dark cabin. My anxiety was through the roof, out of dope and 4+ brutal days from Miami thanks to the return time change. I should have been enjoying my high, but all I could think about was the impending withdrawal. That turned out to be a gross understatement.

The Seattle to Anchorage flight is about 3 hours 45 minutes. Around two hours in, I started feeling the first signs of withdrawal, which always begins with sweating for me. But that couldn't be right - I had just done four bags a few hours earlier.

Maybe it was the altitude, or weak dope, or perhaps I had just skyrocketed my tolerance. Many thoughts and scenarios raced through my head, but the bottom line was I had to stop this oncoming sickness at all costs. There would be no miracles, and it was becoming crystal clear Suboxone was my only hope.

Now, if you take Suboxone too soon before full-blown withdrawal, it throws you into precipitated withdrawal -

the most violent sickness you'll ever experience. It's horrendous. But remember, I'm good at running numbers, here was my logic:

For heavy heroin users like me, withdrawal usually starts around 12 hours after your last dose. Fuck "usually" though - I was going with 12 hours, no question. It had only been three hours since my last bags, but I was already sweating and nauseous.

Must have been weak dope making me sick so soon, I convinced myself. What other explanation could there be?

By my math, three hours was damn close to 12 hours. I was already feeling like shit, and if I just tore the Suboxone strip in half, there was no way I'd send myself into precipitated withdrawal.

There's an official timeline for inducing Suboxone, and you're really supposed to have 6-8 withdrawal symptoms before taking 8mg. I only had two symptoms, but that was close enough for me. Plus, I was only taking 4mg, and I figured I'd seamlessly eliminate the withdrawal.

I put the half strip under my tongue and started bargaining with God.

About an hour and a half out of Anchorage, I started feeling better. Holy shit, I thought - I pulled it off! My anxiety and nausea seemed to be fading. I had no clue what the next 25 minutes had in store.

Precipitated withdrawal ALWAYS hits you 30 minutes on the dot after dosing Suboxone too early. Like flipping a switch, you're suddenly in one of the most violent withdrawals imaginable.

Like clockwork, I started sweating profusely 30 minutes later - not like before when I had thought it was mild withdrawal. No, I looked like I had just come in from a monsoon. This could not be happening, not at 33,000 feet in first class...

Minutes later, I noticed other passengers in first class staring at me. I wondered what they must have been thinking.

How the hell was I going to projectile vomit with no one hearing, seeing or figuring it out? And my wife was right next to me, our elbows touching. I couldn't bolt for the bathroom because I might wake her, and one look at me would give it all away.

Think, think. Okay, the airsick bag in the seat pocket - that was my only option.

I slowly pulled the bag out, draped my jacket over my head, and violently yet quietly hurled into it. You have no idea how hard it is to silently projectile vomit.

Now we were less than an hour from Anchorage, and in 20 or 30 minutes the captain would be flipping on the cabin lights to announce our descent. Please God, don't let me puke in bright light...

Fuck, another wave of nausea. My airsick bag was already half full, and I prayed I wouldn't overflow it. Once again, I attempted to stealthily expel my guts out. This one was much more violent, and I was sure someone had noticed. I just hoped it wasn't my wife.

I Married A Junkie – The Final Chapter

I lowered my makeshift hood and found myself face-to-face with the first-class flight attendant.

I wiped my mouth and whispered, "Yes?"

She replied at full volume, "Sir, are you alright? Do we need to have a medical team waiting at the gate?"

I tried to shush her so my wife wouldn't wake up. I explained I must have gotten food poisoning from some bad sushi in Seattle. Thankfully she bought that and returned to the front galley.

I was royally fucked. My barf bag was full, and I had no idea what to do with it. The lights would be coming on any minute, and my wife would wake up as we got ready to land.

Desperate times call for desperate measures, and another wave was about to hit me. I had maybe 20 seconds to figure something out before I projectile vomited all over myself and the bulkhead.

Full barf bag, 15 seconds. Fuck. I cinched the top of the bag and stuffed it under the seat.

10 seconds. Oh God, the inflight magazine - that was it.

Five seconds. I ripped the magazine open.

Two seconds. I turned toward the window...

One second...

Time was up. I was back to violently puking, but this time into a magazine as I sat in the first-class window seat.

The cabin lights suddenly flipped on, my wife woke up, and I froze in complete horror, still facing the window.

I slowly closed the soaked magazine, praying nothing would seep out, just as my wife asked, "Whatchya doing?"

I replied, "Oh nothing, just admiring the stunning Alaskan landscape and flipping through a magazine."

This haunts me to this day - I gingerly placed the magazine back in the seat pocket and kicked the airsick bag a bit further under the seat.

I've always hoped the cleanup crew found both, because I seriously pity the poor bastard who picked up that magazine on the next flight.

Suggested Listen: Heroin by Badflower

2
Cali

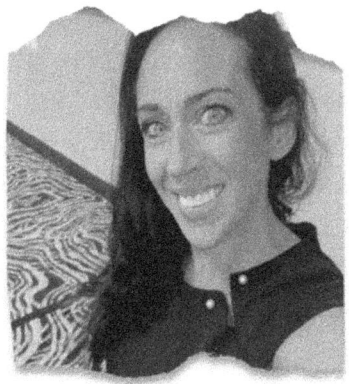

The Alaska trip was supposed to be a makeup for the first disastrous bucket list trip described in the first book. If you remember, by the time we landed in Seattle from Alaska on that trip, Tim was detoxing.

We then drove across the country from Seattle to Idaho, to Montana, down into Wyoming and Denver, and it was miserable. This Alaska trip was meant to redeem that ruined bucket list experience.

The difference this time was we were flying to Seattle for two nights to catch a Cowboys game and have dinner with friends before heading to Alaska for a few days. By the time we landed in Alaska at 1:00 AM, Tim was in full-blown withdrawal. My hopes for a fun-filled trip were dashed.

As we went to get the car, I marveled at Alaska's beauty in late summer, when it's sunny more than dark - even at 1:00 AM, it was still twilight.

All Tim could do was complain about the cold and rush me to get moving. At the hotel, he immediately grabbed all the covers and went to bed, leaving me to unpack everything and shower. By the time I laid down around 3:00 AM, he was already sweating profusely and fidgeting with restless leg syndrome.

I hated this part of his detox because I could never sleep next to him.

This is what caused us to start sleeping in separate bedrooms years ago. He would be sweaty and flop around like a fish. Given my own trouble sleeping due to an overactive mind, I found it impossible to rest. I asked him to take his blanket and pillow to the floor, but he refused.

When he was detoxing, Tim never cared about anyone except himself. Never mind that I paid for this whole trip, again, I still ended up on the floor with my blanket and pillow.

By morning, I was pissed. He was ruining another trip.

Hawaii, St Maarten, Vegas, Bahamas, Puerta Vallarta, The Keys, California, pretty much every trip I could think of at that moment he would detox on and want to leave early to get his fix.

In fact, he left me on several trips to come home and get high.

I went down for breakfast alone, still fuming, got us packed up, and we headed south to Seward to catch a boat for ocean wildlife viewing. I vowed this was the last trip I would pay for since he was such a mess to deal with on a trip.

Once we got to the boat, Tim was freezing and complaining. On the rocking boat, he became sick, spending most of the time in the bathroom or with his hoodie up, head down on the table, refusing to leave the cabin. Meanwhile, I was outside marveling at the whales (including a rare sighting) and glaciers. For two and a half hours, I essentially experienced the trip alone.

This bothered me at first, but it's what ultimately led me to become comfortable traveling solo. Many people say eating alone, traveling alone, or going to a movie alone is empowering. Initially, it didn't feel that way to me, but eventually, I learned to do these things on my own because I grew tired of dragging around an active drug user.

It's like being a babysitter for a toddler that needs constant supervision and oversight and has thrown themselves on the floor, refusing to participate in any activities.

The trip consisted of three days of absolute misery before we flew back to Miami. By the time we returned, I was thoroughly irritated and frustrated. For the first time, I seriously considered my options, realizing I was in an unhappy relationship.

Little did I know, I was in for a real challenge over the next few years.

Suggested Listen: Pissed by Saliva

3
Tim

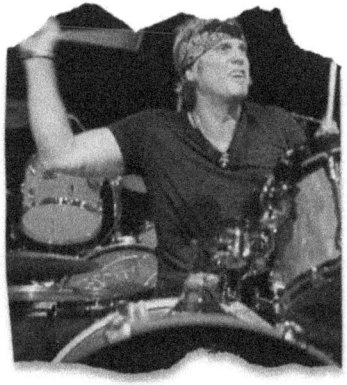

I knew Cali wasn't very happy with me after Alaska. I wanted nothing more than to be totally sober, but I felt I just needed a reason to do it. As if my life, my kids, and my marriage weren't good reasons, I wanted more. That is the thing about addiction, the brain always wants more, and we all know my brain has no shut off valve.

I made myself a deal, if I would get back on national stages, I would get clean, really clean this time. I was able to do it. Cali was so proud of me, and I had never seen her so happy in years. I was proud of myself too. But then the usual boredom and addictive mindset crept in.

I am a touring musician and had completely cleaned up for a US tour that my band was on. The tour was a little over forty days in length, and when I arrived home, I was completely heroin-free. Now, as we opiate addicts know, just because we get clean doesn't mean we stay clean. The very first day that I was home from my tour, I went back to my same dope dealer and purchased my usual ten bags of heroin. But I had a plan. Remember, my brilliant plans? I was going to microdose heroin.

And we all know my brilliant plans always work out, right? This one couldn't have gone much worse.

When I was using heroin daily, I would purchase ten bags of heroin in the morning and snort three at a time just to "get right." Then a few more at a time throughout the day, and I would need to make a return trip to Liberty City, just before bed.

Here I am, forty-one days clean from all opiates, with ten bags of heroin, a loaded gun (we will get to that whole story later, just remember it's my Bahamian Buddies), and a brand-new BMW leaving Liberty City.

What could go wrong?

A couple of things happened next. First, I used my typical three bags at a time after being clean for forty-one days. Second, I was targeted leaving Liberty City by people that wanted my BMW for a ring of smash and grab jewelry heists that were going around. They watched my heroin transaction. They knew as well as I did that I wasn't waiting until I got home to get high.

In true fashion they watched me snort the first three bags off the front of my phone, and they followed me out of the dope hole for a few miles and pulled in front of me and did the old "brake at a green light" trick, hoping I would be high and tap them from behind, which I predictably did.

I Married A Junkie – The Final Chapter

I got out and apologized, thinking it was my fault, and they said, "No problem, man. Just follow us to the little bodega up the street and take $100 out of the ATM, and we won't call the cops." They knew I would "bite" since I was probably high and had more dope in the car, which I predictably did, and they didn't even know about the loaded gun under the front seat.

And third, I was in the beginning stages of a total overdose from being completely clean and using three bags of heroin at a time, initially. These three factors created the complete shit show that was to follow.

By the time both cars got to the bodega, which was less than five minutes away, I could barely walk, and I had a bad habit of leaving the key fob to my new BMW in the center cup holder. One of the predators took me inside the bodega for his $100 while the other went directly for my car.

The last thing I remember was putting my debit card into the ATM and not being able to remember my pin. Then I completely collapsed on the bodega floor. Once they realized I was "out" and the key fob was in the car, their work became a whole lot easier, even without their $100. The bodega owner called 911, and the car thieves took off in my car.

The next thing I remember is waking up in the back of a moving ambulance. When you are in a bodega one minute and waking up in the back of a moving ambulance in what appears to be the next moment, it can be startling and downright confusing. After being administered Narcan and coming to, the paramedics began asking me questions to verify my well-being. They first asked my name, which I answered correctly. Next, they asked who the President of the United States was, which I answered correctly. Then finally, they asked if I knew where I was.

Remember, I mentioned just coming off a US tour? Well, the tour ended a few days before this incident, and we played Dallas, Texas, two weeks into the forty-day tour. I had not been to Dallas in over three weeks.

However, my answer to their final question was, "I am in Dallas on tour with my band, and I think I scored bad dope after the show." The medics informed me that I was not in Dallas and had overdosed on heroin in Miami.

After that answer, there was no sign of any refusal of medical treatment. I was going right to the nearest hospital for further observation. As hard as I tried to sign myself out, the doctor made me sit with an IV for a few hours until he felt I was safe to leave.

Now mind you, I love to be barefoot, I had my sandals off in the car, and I had to walk back to the bodega where I thought my car was barefoot. And not being 100% mentally awake yet, it took a few hours to walk back and find the bodega.

I walked in, and the guy behind the counter came around, gave me a huge hug, and said, "Sir, I thought you were dead! I am the one who dragged you outside and called 911."

I thanked him and asked him where my car was. He replied with, "What car"

I Married A Junkie – The Final Chapter

Now I am in trouble. My car was nowhere to be found, and I hadn't answered my phone for hours. My wife was panicked, not to mention extremely angry.

Thankfully I had my phone on me when I collapsed, since my thoughtful wife had bought the credit card holder that sticks to the back of your phone because I kept leaving my wallet everywhere I went and losing it.

I hadn't answered my phone in hours. Thirty-three missed calls from the wife. My brilliant plan was feeling a lot less brilliant and more destructive at this point. What can I do?

I weighed my options and did what any married man would do in my position. I made up a story and called her. I told her and the police that I ran into a local gas station for a Monster and left my car unlocked and running. I told them when I came back out, the car was gone. I made numerous mistakes that day that almost killed me, but so did the car thieves.

First, never steal a new BMW. They all have LoJack GPS location devices on them. Once we reported it stolen, they had the exact location within ten minutes.

Second, if you are going to steal a car, look under the front seat and throughout the car for things that you might not want in there if you get caught.

And lastly, don't park a brand-new BMW that you just stole right in front of your own apartment. The police sat on my car until one of the car thieves came downstairs and tried to drive off. They rushed the car and arrested him.

The police called me to tell me that my car was safe and sound, and the car thief was under arrest. The cop then said, "I'm assuming the loaded gun and seven bags of heroin that we found in the car aren't yours."

I replied with, "No, sir. I don't own a gun, and I don't do heroin." The gun wasn't registered to me, and I sure wasn't claiming any heroin.

Not only did the car thief get a grand theft auto charge, but he also got possession of a concealed firearm by a convicted felon and a heroin charge.

Was that right on my part? Probably not, but neither was stealing my car! I found out days later from my dealer that he watched the car follow me out of the dope hole and described it to me, and it matched exactly with the car I bumped into. That's when it sank in that I had been followed and set up by these car thieves.

Now, I wasn't a total heartless asshole. I was asked to come to the station to ID the guy for the gun charge.

In my state, that is a mandatory three-year sentence to run consecutively with any other sentence they receive. I refused to cooperate on that charge only, and he was charged with grand theft auto and possession of heroin.

The heroin charge was my gift to him for stealing my car.

As you can see, our addictive minds can get us in a world of trouble in a matter of minutes. Not to mention, I had almost ended my life and my marriage that day.

I Married A Junkie – The Final Chapter

Suggested Listen: *Devil by Shinedown*

Dr. Cali Estes & Tim Estes

4
Cali

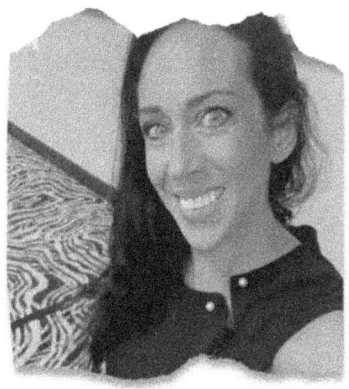

Tim loved fancy and shiny things, especially cars. Being raised as a 'tom boy' and working on cars with my dad, I loved cars, especially anything with some horsepower. I convinced Tim to get his first Hemi. Probably not smart on my part, but I loved stick shift cars and power and well, I could drive it too. When Dodge (I am a Mopar girl) released the Dodge Challenger, I wanted one. I wanted the Hellcat, but I thought let's start with the SRT.

Off we went to the dealership and bought a neon green SRT Dodge Challenger. We kept it parked at the RV park with Tim's tour bus or "Crow's Nest" as the band called it. I had also bought my 7th Jeep Wrangler at the time, The Beast, a Rubicon stick shift, white with cranberry interior. Some girls buy clothes and make-up, I buy cars and shoes! It would be cheaper to buy expensive purses and own a Sephora store at this point.

We had that car for only 3 months, before Tim crashed it while high on heroin. He hid the car, thinking I wouldn't see the front-end damage. I was furious, I made him fix it himself.

I was done enabling him and fixing all his problems. He had to come up with the cash to fix the hood and quarter panels. He fixed the car and then wanted to get one level up - a Go Mango Dodge Challenger Scat Pack, which has even more horsepower than the SRT.

The only reason I agreed was because I love cars, especially rare stick shifts like this 2018 model. I also told him he would have to have six months clean before I bought any more cars, and I would drug test him. Through another brutal detox he went. Vomiting, night sweats, headache, restless legs and more. Since he was able to pull it off, I bought the car.

He did well with the Scat Pack for a while. Then one day I got a phone call.

The phone rang. It was Tim, out of breath. "I ran out of gas and need you to bring me some. I'm too far from a gas station."

I took a deep breath, thinking, "Here we go again." I didn't understand how he was always running out of gas everywhere we went. This was a Hemi engine that needed to be fueled regularly. Letting it run bone dry would cause problems.

"He can't be this stupid," I muttered under my breath as I grabbed the reserve gas can, filled it up, and brought it to him.

He wouldn't tell me his location until I assured him that I was on my way with the gas. Finally, he admitted he was on the side of the entrance ramp to I-95, having passed two gas stations. He was obviously heading to buy drugs with whatever money he had when he ran out of fuel.

I brought him the gas, completely pissed off. I didn't understand how he could treat a nice, $70,000 souped-up car like garbage. It felt like red flag after red flag that I kept missing because I didn't want to admit I had no control over the situation. My husband was deep in addiction, and everything else, including me, was less important.

Even our property and the things I worked hard to provide meant nothing to him. When someone is actively using, no matter what you do or provide, they will disregard it because their main concern is themselves.

They are incredibly selfish individuals when in the throes of addiction. Still, I had hoped I could somehow fix the situation. He had just had 6 months clean time and here we are...again. I felt like I was on a merry go round, and at this point I was ready to jump off. But maybe, just maybe he could get it together.

Looking back, I really wish I had a strong friend to wake me up and tell me I wasn't going to be able to fix him, that nothing I did or said could change his behavior. Even with his brief periods of sobriety, he never really got his act together.

I put the gas in the car, and off he went. About an hour later, he called saying the car wouldn't start. I assumed he had already burned through the $5 of gas without filling the tank further.

He wouldn't tell me where he was, just that he was using my AAA card to tow the car to the dealership in Hollywood. I arrived in time to watch a tow truck driver completely dump the front end of my car off the lift. He didn't use a flatbed tow, which he should have, and Tim didn't even notice.

The next day the dealership called and sure enough, the entire engine was shot. This was a heavy-duty, expensive Hemi engine - about $13,000, plus another $2,000 for the installed McLeod clutch. Close to $15,000 in repairs. Along with the tow damage, probably another $10-15,000 in body work. All in, we were looking at around $30,000 to fix this vehicle, and I knew I would be the one footing the bill. I was furious.

I turned to Tim and said, "Here we go again, another vehicle you've wrecked or destroyed."

He swore he didn't do anything, that the engine just blew, trying to convince me it was the same issue I was having with my own 2018 Jeep Wrangler, which was in the process of a lemon law claim due to recurring clutch/transmission failures on the highway.

The following day, the service department called to inform me the Scat Pack hadn't had an oil change, ever.

I Married A Junkie – The Final Chapter

We had put almost 50,000 miles on it from Tim driving all over and he never once thought to change the oil.

When someone is active in their addiction, they don't think of anything but themselves. I had given him the credit card multiple times to get the oil changed, but I couldn't monitor his every move.

In a normal relationship, partners handle various responsibilities - vehicle maintenance, making sure there's food in the house, etc. But all of this fell on me. I was doing every job and getting none of the benefits.

Managing and running a national company, flying to see clients, helping with his band, and handling all of the financial responsibilities took its toll on me.

I'm sure on social media my life looked amazing because Tim would post about his incredible wife, but in reality, I was living in hell. I did everything I could to help him, and he couldn't even help himself.

Out of the 19 cars we owned, he destroyed or ruined 18 of them. The only one he didn't was my diesel Jeep Wrangler that I wouldn't let him drive. He was a loose cannon, a runaway train going off the tracks and nothing I did or said would change it.

Suggested Listen:
Runaway Train by Soul Asylum

5
Tim

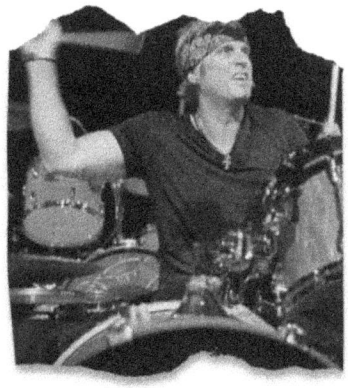

After I blew the Dodge Challenger Scat Pack, Cali told me that I had to get clean and get a job. A real job, not just playing drums. When we met, I was a touring musician, but I also did electrical work to pay the bills.

I figured two things out that day. I would quit opiates and go back to electrical work. Now I NEED to concentrate, because I am dealing with low voltage electrical wires, and I can get shocked pretty easy.

Sometimes just for fun in Manhattan, Johnny (my old singer from my band The Deadlyz and I would just shock each other for fun on the job. One of us would be 8 ft up on a ladder and the other would crawl up silently and shock him with something. It was fun, probably not the safest thing to do, but hey I have ADHD and well, PINK SQUIRREL!!!

My brilliant plan (remember how all my plans are brilliant) is to quit opiates and go back to using cocaine. Let me explain. Using cocaine helps me concentrate and I am easily distracted. I am at my best when I am doing multiple things at once. I thrive in a commercial kitchen cooking multiple orders at once while putting together food order tickets with multiple items from different sections of the kitchen line. And I thrive doing this while communicating with 10 different food servers. This was only a portion of time in my life.

I also thrive doing electrical work, which involves 6 to 10 different wire sizes going in 6 to 10 different rooms, and this is done in 3 to four different houses being wired in one day. Do you see the pattern yet? If not, you will after this. My life passion is playing and touring in a rock band playing, you guessed it, DRUMS!

I am at my best playing because you need to play different things at once, with both hands and feet. If you have ever seen me play, you know I am a VERY VISUAL drummer! Not to mention, the drummer leads the band in tempo and timing. I was a master at doing many multiple things at once and thriving at them.

I also learned at the age of 18 that using cocaine seemed to bring it all together on a concentration level. Yes, cocaine seemed to help me concentrate. Now, I am obviously not a doctor, but cocaine seems to mimic the effects of Adderall. And users of Adderall compare the effects of it to cocaine at times, especially those who use Adderall that do NOT suffer from ADHD.

I Married A Junkie – The Final Chapter

It seems almost simple to understand, yet it seems to pass right over my head when thinking about it. Would it be safe to say that there is a connection between those who "suffer" from ADHD and those same people being able to thrive in chaotic scenarios where they are required to do multiple things at once?

And would it be fair to say that both Adderall and cocaine could help these very same people concentrate when doing these tasks that require major multitasking? I know what my answer would be, hence why doctors doll out Adderall like candy.

I am also aware of what the legal ramifications of using cocaine have caused me and my family in the past. I remind myself that I have 24 felonies and 14 misdemeanors but then my addicted mind convinces me of this: cocaine use can become addictive and usually always does, just like all the beer at my local grocery store.

Or just like all those donuts at my local bakery or the slot machines at my local casino. And especially as addictive as all those cigarettes at every gas station and grocery store in my city. I tell myself I can stop when I want to as I buy an 8 Ball and head to my new electrical job.

Suggested Listen: *Retox by The Deadlyz*

Need for pleasure
I've got the secret, blow your plans off
I've got the ticket, need for craving
I've got the punchline, take your hats off
I've got the ticket

Starstruck, starstruck
Stage and lights
Starstruck, starstruck
Stage is life

Retox, baby
Retox, baby
Another line down
Another line down

Retox, baby
Retox, baby
Another line down
Another line down

Locked and loaded
Trigger an explosion, settle for nothing
I've got the rocket, your tunnels achin'
My pistol's shakin', take your pants off
I've got the ticket

Starstruck, starstruck
Stage and lights
Starstruck, starstruck
Stage is life

Retox, baby
Retox, baby
Another line down
Another line down

Retox, baby
Retox, baby
Another line down
Another line down

I gotta get high
I gotta get high now
Another line
Another line down

Retox, baby
Retox, baby
Another line down
Another line down

Take it slow
It has to stop sometime
No more getting high
No more

We leave behind baby
Retox, baby
Another line down
Another line down

Retox, baby
Retox, baby
Another line down
Another line down

Songwriter: Johnny Moody

Lyrics © Johnny Moody and The Deadlyz 2008

6
Cali

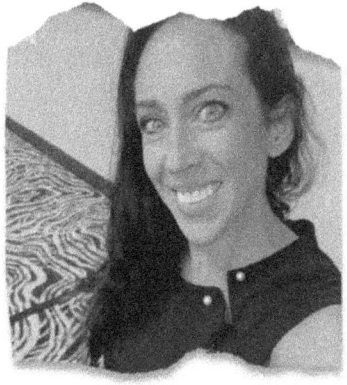

We had just headed down into Brickell, Miami, so I could get adjusted by the chiropractor and visit a few friends for lunch. We had a great lunch, everything seemed normal, and we were heading out in the black pickup truck towards Target to grab some supplies before heading home.

About halfway into Wynwood, the arts district that sits next to Overtown (a rougher area known for gang activity and adjacent to Liberty City, where Tim used to buy drugs), the police suddenly lit us up. We pulled over to the side of the road, and I thought, "I wonder what he did now? Speeding? Taillight out?" I knew it wasn't expired tags because the truck was in my name.

I didn't even get a chance to think. My door was flung open and there were SWAT officers all around the vehicle, pointing semi-automatics at my face and telling me to get out. I stood there for a second thinking, "What the fuck did he do now?" This couldn't be a simple drug possession. My husband's a drug addict, not a dealer, and as far as I knew, he wasn't trafficking drugs across state lines. What could this be?

They put us on the side of the road and literally ripped apart the entire pickup, like I'd seen on TV shows.

They pulled out the seats, knifed them open, pulled out the stuffing. They were obviously looking for something but wouldn't answer when I asked what this was about.

I had to sit there in silence while they tore apart my vehicle, causing thousands of dollars in damage.

About 20 minutes in, one of the officer's mics rang and he was called to his vehicle. He left us with the other SWAT and police officers, on the side of the road. He quickly returned and said, "We got him."

They immediately stopped what they were doing, headed to their vehicles, and took off our handcuffs. I said, "What's going on? Why were we detained, and you ripped apart my vehicle causing thousands in damage? And you're just stranding us here on the side of the road?"

Apparently, it turned out that our exact vehicle - same make, model, and color - was just used in a major jewelry heist in downtown Miami's jewelry district. That pickup was seen leaving the crime scene and heading down the same road we were on. We happened to be about ten car lengths ahead of the actual vehicle. The perpetrators had stolen the vehicle, robbed the jewelry store, then made a turn towards Liberty City, where the cops nabbed them and made the arrests.

This story always stuck with me because for 20 minutes, I was sure my husband had been trafficking drugs, hiding drugs, or doing something completely illegal beyond just using.

I'll never forget, he looked at me and said, "Well, that was fun." I thought to myself, "There was nothing fun about this."

He found it exhilarating, an adrenaline rush, whereas I couldn't believe I was being detained for a vehicle I owned when I had done nothing wrong. They ripped apart my truck and left it in pieces on the side of the road. We had to put the seats back in just to drive it, and they were ruined along with the dash.

The kicker is, you don't have much legal recourse when police search your car because they thought they had probable cause. There's no way they were going to pay for the damage. They literally left us stranded on the roadside with pieces of my vehicle strewn about.

This was the one time I was pissed at my husband, and it wasn't even his fault.

Suggested Listen: Welcome to the Circus by Five Finger Death Punch

7
Tim

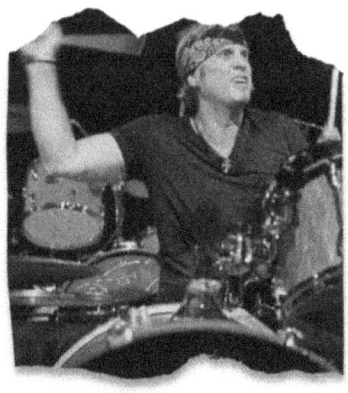

I knew Cali had always wanted a Hellcat, especially after the issue with the Challenger Scat Pack and my forgetting to do oil changes. I figured I'd surprise her with one of my brilliant plans. Remember my brilliant plans? Here goes.

While Cali was looking at buying another Wrangler - she wanted a stick shift Rubicon, and we'd found the perfect one - I was scouring the country for Hellcats. I told myself I wouldn't buy one unless it was neon green or "Go Green" as they call it, like my first SRT that I accidentally ran into another car when I nodded out. I know it is a sore subject with Cali because these are two nice muscle cars that I destroyed; I just want to make this right for her.

After searching for about two days, I found the perfect Hellcat at the right price. I called and set it up, thinking it would be a great surprise for her. I told Cali I was heading to Georgia and would be back the same day.

My brilliant plan was to get to the airport early, hop on a plane, and get to the dealership. I pre-negotiated with them to pick me up at the airport as soon as I landed, whisk me to the dealership, and have all the paperwork ready for me to sign. I even sent them my driver's license and everything they'd need ahead of time to make it flawless and easy. I could hop in the Hellcat, fuel up, and head home. It's a nine-hour drive, but with a bump here and there, I knew I could do it in seven.

I called Cali when I got to the airport, figuring I had a full day because she was going to work, hit the gym, and do her normal routine. Everything went according to plan - I landed, they picked me up flawlessly, I secured the car, and I was headed back.

The one key thing I didn't tell her, and wasn't planning to until we got back, was that I might have put the car charge on her unlimited American Express credit card. But I figured once she saw the car, she'd forgive me. My whole plan was "do now, ask for forgiveness later," which had worked so far in our marriage. I thought this couldn't go wrong either.

The car was as beautiful as I'd imagined - big slick tires and 797 horsepower (or more, they weren't exactly sure) under the hood. It was a Redeye, and I was pretty pleased with my decision.

I made it home in just under eight hours and pulled into the parking lot, excited to see Cali's reaction. I figured she'd give me a big hug and kiss on the cheek for buying us such a cool car. In true Cali fashion, though, she was pissed off that I'd put $65,000 on a credit card without asking. But hey, we're married, and in Florida, half of everything is mine. I figured it wasn't a big deal. I'd find a way to pay it back.

That's another one of my brilliant plans - promising to pay things back but getting distracted by new shiny objects like the RV or the new pickup truck, and just kind of forgetting I was supposed to be making monthly payments. But hey, right now I have a beautiful Hellcat. She was going to love it, and everything would be fine, right?

Well, I hoped it would be.

Suggested Listen: [Say Fuck It by Buckcherry](#)

8
Cali

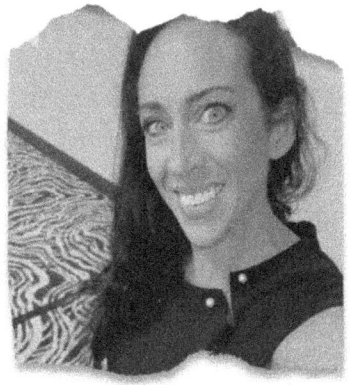

I remember his buying the Hellcat a bit differently.

The phone rang as I was standing in the driveway about to get into my Jeep Wrangler and go to the gym. It was Tim, calling with a lot of background noise. He said he was at the airport, headed to Atlanta to pick something up, and would be back tonight or tomorrow.

It's not unusual for people struggling with substance abuse to do something reckless, but it is unusual for them to announce it beforehand. This was a first for me. He was calling to tell me what he was about to do before doing it.

I ran through every scenario in my head of why he could be going to Atlanta. He used to have friends there he would visit and play music with, and even an ex-girlfriend. He was sober and had over a year under his belt, I figured it can't be that reckless.

He hung up, and when I tried to call back, it went to voicemail. He texted that his plane was taking off and he'd call me later, then turned his phone off again. It's not unusual for someone in active addiction to shut their phone off, but it is odd for them to inform you first. They usually act first and ask for forgiveness later.

I was not used to a sober version of Tim again and was just settling in to enjoying the way he was when I met him. I had to remind myself that a sober Tim was impulsive as hell.

About five hours later, he called, super excited. "Hey babe, you're never going to guess what I have!"

I replied, "Well, it's been about five hours. You should be in Georgia by now." He confirmed he was and that "they" picked him up at the airport and took him straight to the dealership.

"Dealership? What are you doing?" I asked.

He told me to listen, and I heard a powerful engine revving in the background. "I'm not just looking at it... I think I may have purchased it," he said.

My blood started to boil. He had just bought a car somewhere in Georgia, and we didn't need another car. We already had four in the driveway, plus an RV his son was living in and a pickup truck I paid for that his son drove.

He came back on the phone saying, "You're going to love this. It's beautiful."

I retorted, "Well, unless you're buying a Hellcat, I really don't want to know."

I Married A Junkie – The Final Chapter

He simply said, "Then I'll see you in a couple hours," and hung up.

I was really upset, wondering what he could have possibly bought in Atlanta of all places. He was obviously driving it back home to Miami, probably a nine-hour drive or more.

An hour later, I tried calling back, but his phone was off. He didn't want to tell me what it was - I would have to be surprised.

Being surprised as Tim's wife was nothing new. He would do crazy, spontaneous things all the time, from buying an RV on a whim to taking last-minute trips to Vegas. It could be fun, except for the fact that I always ended up having to pay for everything.

Fast forward - I finished work, went to the gym, walked and fed the dogs, showered and got ready for bed.

He finally called, saying he had two hours left to drive and was starting to fall asleep. He wanted me to talk to him so he could safely bring home whatever he just bought. It was midnight.

I brewed a fresh pot of coffee and talked to him for the next two hours until he pulled into the driveway around 2am.

I heard it before I saw it.

He was flying high on energy drinks, having been up all night. He pulled up in the most beautiful neon green and black Hellcat Redeye you've ever seen. Stick shift, of course. I took it for a spin - it was gorgeous.

But then I had to ask, "How did you buy this? You don't have a job. Is this something I'm going to have to pay for?"

He claimed it was already paid for, that he just "threw it on the credit card" - my business Amex with no limit.

Now I had a $65,000 Hellcat Red Eye in the business name that I would probably rarely drive, but it made him happy. If he wanted something, he would just buy it, and I'd end up paying for it.

The good news was I owned it free and clear, and it was a Limited Edition. It would only increase in value.

The sad part was, about six months later he crashed it while trying to detox from opiates (again) on his way to band practice. He fell asleep at the wheel on detox meds and rear-ended a truck going 65mph.

Suggested Listen:
<u>*Accidents Can Happen by Sixx: A.M.*</u>

9
Tim

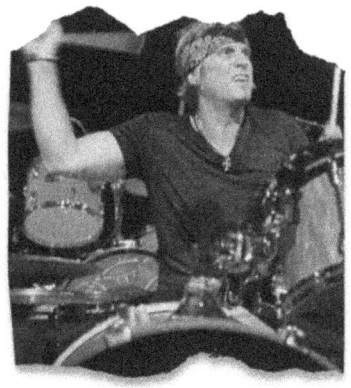

I know I keep repeating this, but crazy shit runs through my head when using heroin, and this might be the craziest one.

It's next to impossible to finance a massive heroin habit unless you are making a mid-six-figure salary or selling drugs yourself. At this point in my life, I was doing neither. I needed another minor adjustment (remember my adjustments from the first chapter?)

Making a mid-six-figure salary would take time, and that's time I do not have. My habit has re-escalated more than it's ever been. And selling heroin is just asking for a lengthy prison sentence. Plus, I've already been to prison twice, I would get major time. What can I do?

I know! Denver has always been good to me, and weed is legal in Denver. Here's another one of my brilliant plans. Let's buy real estate in Denver, invest a few grand in material, grow some weed, and drive it back to Miami to sell it. It is totally legal to grow in Denver and I know just the person to teach me out there!

If I get caught, which will never happen, I will get a slap on the wrist for a weed charge in Miami. With the massive income I will then have, I will be able to pull my weight financially and finance my massive heroin habit.

Less than a year later, I own property in Denver with a legal cannabis growing operation. How did I learn to grow weed in less than a year when I knew nothing about it?

Well, one source must remain anonymous, and the other was my Bahamian buddy (remember the gun in my BMW?) He was a weed expert and taught me a lot. This plan was perfect. Except for one small problem. A few months later, it was time to leave Miami and go harvest our first load.

Of course, I need dope for the trip, so it's off to Liberty City. Now, this is the first and only time this has ever happened to me. Miami Police were everywhere in the dope hole, and The First 48 film crew were there.

There wasn't a soul answering their phones or on the corner. Great. A fucking murder is shutting the neighborhood down. Time for one of my minor adjustments (these all work well for me).

I call my Bahamian buddy who will be traveling with me and ask if he can score heroin. He says no, but that he can get thirty-milligram Roxies.

Okay, we are going to be in Denver for about a month and then make the three-day drive from Denver to Miami.

I started running numbers again. Fuck it, I want them all! I picked him up with over a hundred Roxies (he was fronting me), and we started driving to Denver.

What a stress-free trip that was. A few Roxies every now and then. We stopped and got a hotel when we were tired, and in three and a half days, we made it to Denver.

Everything seemed perfect, except Roxies metabolize and leave your opiate receptors much quicker than heroin or fentanyl. This means you need more sooner than other opiates.

Obviously, my Bahamian buddy wouldn't let me hold the pills. It seemed like every thirty minutes; I was asking for three more. He had unlimited weed, and it was legal. He wasn't even counting how many I was using. I've never seen a man tear up by seeing massive amounts of weed like my Bahamian buddy did. It was moving.

After about two weeks, we were done with the harvest, trimming, and packaging of around twenty pounds of quality weed. We were supposed to stay a month because that would put us at the exact midway point of Thanksgiving and Christmas for the three-and-a-half-day drive back to Miami. And this seemed to be the safest time to drive twenty pounds of weed cross-country, in my opinion.

Well, our work in Denver is done, and all we need to do now is relax for two weeks and do three more Roxies. Except my Bahamian buddy just informed me that I only had ten remaining. Ten Roxies for fourteen days? That's not going to work.

These minor adjustments are going to be the death of me. Obviously, I need to get back to Miami, and quickly. Ten Roxies will barely get me to Kansas City with hotel stops. Plus, being in Denver, while packaging twenty pounds of weed, is my favorite time and place to do Roxies. If you read or listened to the previous chapter, you know how this story goes. I tell my Bahamian buddy that we are leaving tonight.

"Tonight? Are you fucking kidding me? We need another week or so to come up with how we are going to pack the car," says my buddy.

I'm way ahead of him. A few months ago, I flew to LA and bought a drum set from a well-known rock drummer. I had it shipped to my place in Denver. Here's my plan. We are going to take all the drum heads off, pack the bass drum and every tom with twenty pounds of weed and pack the car with drums. Perfect plan. We will never get pulled over.

Except we are driving a BMW X3, with Florida tags, I have a Miami driver's license, our route is Denver to Miami, and in my passenger seat is a Bahamian with long dreads and gold teeth. What could possibly go wrong?

With the altitude, Denver in late November is very cold. Warmer weather wasn't even a factor to me, but it will be soon. With absolutely no sleep, we set out for Miami at eleven o'clock pm with twenty pounds of weed stuffed in my drums.

Suggested Listen:
Face Down in the Dirt by Mötley Crüe

10
Tim

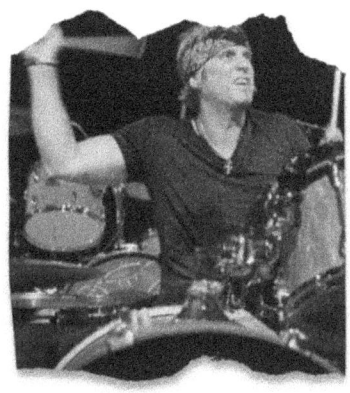

Picture this: me driving with my Bahamian friend beside me, my 5-piece drum kit stuffed full of marijuana. Growing weed in Denver was totally legal but driving it clear across the country was probably not my best idea ever. Especially since I forgot that as we headed south, things would heat up.

As you can imagine, the car started to get hot. I hadn't packed the drums well with any buffer, the smell became almost unbearable.

Sure enough, somewhere near the end of Kansas, a cop lit up behind me. I looked at my Bahamian friend and thought, "I am not going to jail today. This is not going to happen."

But of course, my addicted mind raced through every scenario.

Surprisingly, my main concern wasn't jail time or being separated from my family. My only thought was getting to Miami for more Roxies before I started detoxing on this trip. Now my addicted mind started thinking of how I was going to convince this officer that we were simply passing through on the way to a gig.

When the cop pulled us over, the entire car reeked of weed. He asked what we were doing, and we said we were visiting Denver. Then, of course, he wanted to search the car. I thought we were completely, 100% screwed.

Every worst-case scenario ran through my head - from getting the car impounded to going to jail, to what I'd tell my wife. She didn't even know about this; she thought I was visiting my son for a couple of weeks.

But as things often do for me, it worked out.

The cop said, "I'm going to let you go, but I want you to open up the drums, open the bags of weed, and dump them out on the side of the road."

I was relieved we weren't getting in trouble, thinking I could still get home and get Roxies and heroin as quickly as possible. My Bahamian buddy, though, looked devastated. He couldn't believe we were about to abandon several pounds of marijuana on the roadside.

I opened my drums and dumped everything out, watching as the cop lit it on fire. I thought, "There goes my instant money, my habit, my way to finance myself."

Two weeks out here, plus driving time, and I still had to get home and score opiates. Everything we'd worked for was gone. But my addicted brain shut down those thoughts and focused solely on getting home and getting high.

We got back in the car and barreled down the road at about 110 miles an hour, trying to reach Miami before the onset of withdrawal symptoms.

I never told Cali what happened because she didn't know why we were out there in the first place. My Bahamian buddy, though, never spoke to me again after this incident.

Suggested Listen: <u>Hurricane by I Prevail</u>

11
Cali

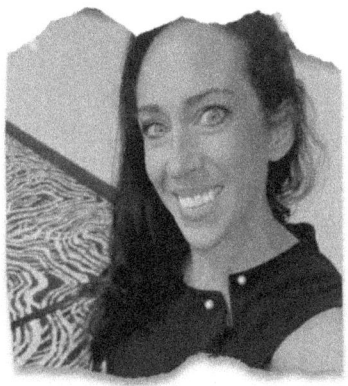

The first day I asked for a divorce was in the year 2019. We were living in Miami in a condo, and we had the tour bus, or the Crow's Nest, as they call it, parked up in Margate at a luxury resort center. We were driving up from Miami to get the bus, get it packed, get it cleaned up, do an oil change, and the band was going to meet us later that night.

We were going to head up to Georgia, spend the night there. They were playing a show the next day, and then we were going to head from there over to Tennessee and Kentucky for a few shows.

On the way up in the car, Tim had a very strange facial expression, and he seemed pained by something. And me, being a typical therapist, I kept saying, "What's wrong? Tell me what's wrong."

I was trying to figure out what the problem was, because as a trained clinical therapist, I always want to get to the why. Why are you behaving this way? Why is there a problem? What's happening? I wanted to get to the root cause of the issue, just like I do with all my clients.

Of course, I ask, "What's going on?"

And I immediately regretted my decision.

He said to me, "You got to promise not to be mad at me."

And whenever he said that I knew he was about to come clean about something stupid that he did.

I said, "I can't promise that anymore. What did you do?" And he wouldn't tell me.

We're pulling into the RV park, which is about a 30-minute drive from Miami, if you know the area. As we were pulling in, he stopped, and I said, "What's wrong with the bus?"

And he goes, "Nothing's wrong with the bus. The bus is fine."

We had a spot way at the back of the park, and it took a little while to get in there, and I was on pins and needles for the drive. I finally was able to see the bus and it looked fine from the outside. He had so many car and truck crashes that nothing surprised me anymore.

As we were getting out of the truck, he said, "Just promise not to be mad at me."

He opened the door, and I walked on the bus, and all the TVs were gone. There's three TVs on the bus. All of them were gone. Just wires and holes hanging around.

I Married A Junkie – The Final Chapter

And I looked at him, and I said, "I want a divorce."

That's all I said. I didn't raise my voice. I didn't get upset. I was done and so over this insane, chaotic behavior.

And he goes, "I don't know what to do. The band is going to be here in two hours."

And I said, "I don't know what to tell you. Where are the TVs?"

And he said, "I had to pawn them because I bought drugs."

Of course he pawned them for drugs. And they became due. Today's the 90-day mark, and if I don't pay for them, we're going to lose them.

He would always pawn something, my jewelry, his tools, his drum set, and then he would pay the interest for the three months. Then when the actual borrowed price was due, he never had the money to pay it. If I wanted them back, like the signed Nikki Sixx bass guitar, I had to buy it back from the pawn shop.

Countless times I had to get his drum equipment out the day of a show, or tools so he could work, even his wedding ring and expensive watch went in there. It got so bad that I had to lock up all my (and his) jewelry and he had to ask me to wear it.

Here we are again, and it falls on me. There are three TVs missing from the RV and the band is coming over in a few hours to get on the bus and travel. What do I tell them? He would always minimize and downplay the cost of his pawning excursions.

I asked, "What's the total?"

He responds, "It's only $300. It's not a big deal. Just give me $300. Give me $200 extra just in case it's a little bit more."

$500 for three TVs that I had already bought and paid for.

Now I'm in a pickle, because if I don't give him the $500 for the three TVs, I'm going to be out even more money. Each TV alone is about $1,000 for that RV, not to mention installation and everything, because I don't know how to do all that. There are wires hanging everywhere.

I ran the math in my head, and I think, okay, $500 solved the problem. The band is on the way over. We had to have TVs to get up there. You're going to have people coming on and off. It's a tour bus. They're going to be signing things and whatnot. Can't look like a ratchet tour bus. We must take care of it.

Of course, I give him the money, and he leaves. He called me from the pawn store, as he always did, and it wasn't $500, as it always isn't.

He said, "You know, I'm so sorry. I got the numbers wrong."

He always got the numbers wrong. Always downplayed and minimized how bad his behavior was. And that was a red flag when it came to addiction. That's what addicts do. They maximize the problem, minimize their behavior in the problem. Take no accountability. The total bill was $1,500.

At this point, the band is calling. They're about 30 minutes out. He's still at the pawn store. The TVs are not up there yet, and they're on their way.

What do I do? I put the money in his account.

In the back of my head, I think, just get through today and things will be okay. That is a mistake a lot of people make when they are the loved one of an addict. It is an enabling behavior. But you stop and go, just do damage control today, figure it out. Today we'll get to the tour, we'll make sure things get better, and I'll make sure he gets detoxed.

I made him promise me that was it. He was stopping.

We are good to go. Sure enough, we get the TVs, put them in, and we take off to tour.

The engine light comes on for the first time. We are driving on our way to Georgia, and the engine light comes on. Not a big deal, except I've got two dogs in the RV, a bunch of stuff, and a whole band full of people and I am the responsible one.

Suggested Listen: Crows by Saliva

I Married A Junkie – The Final Chapter

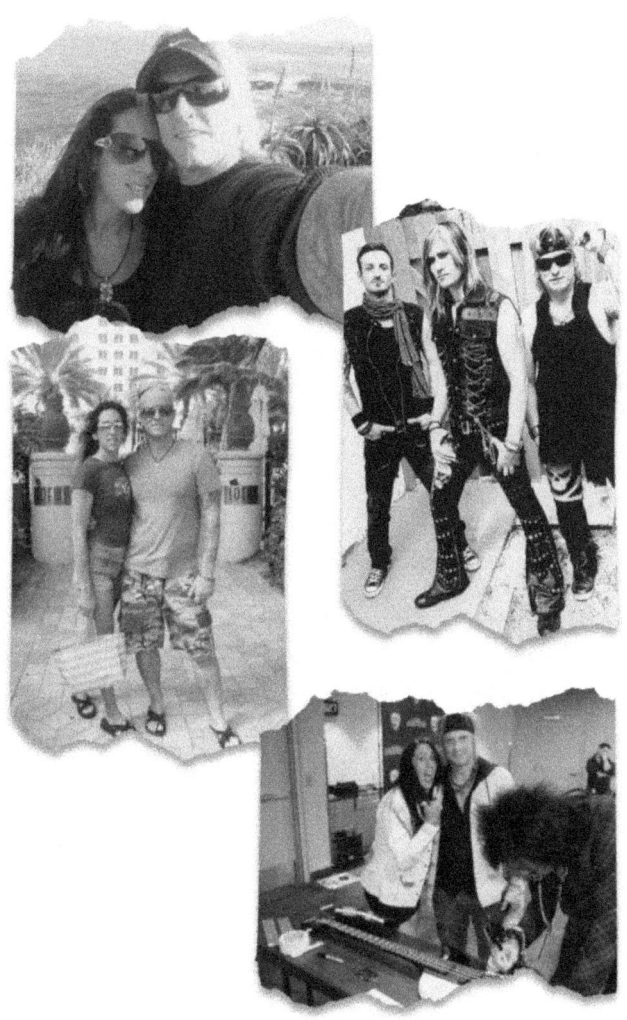

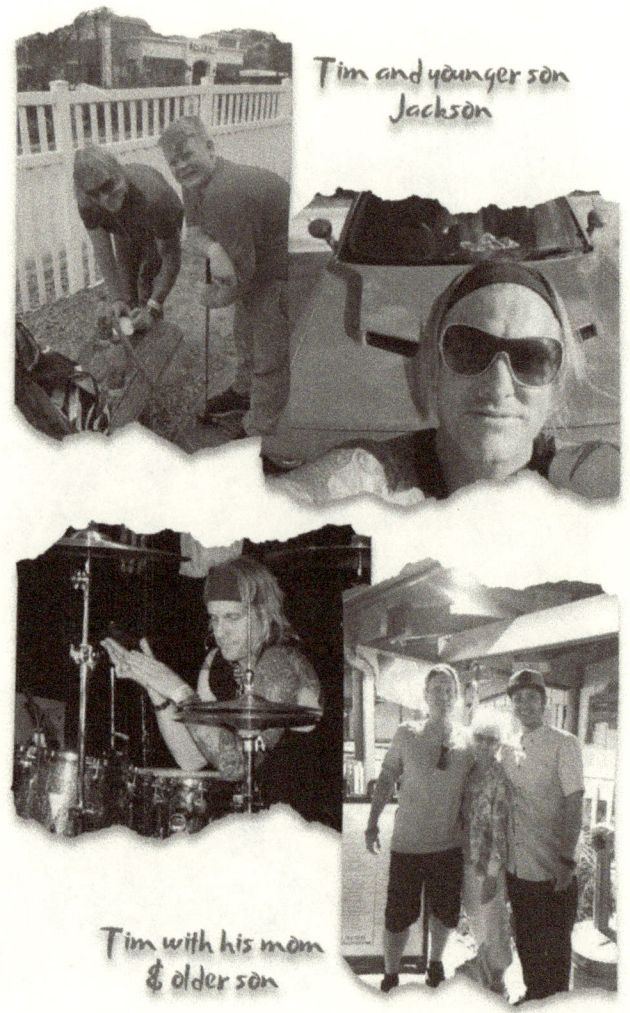

I Married A Junkie – The Final Chapter

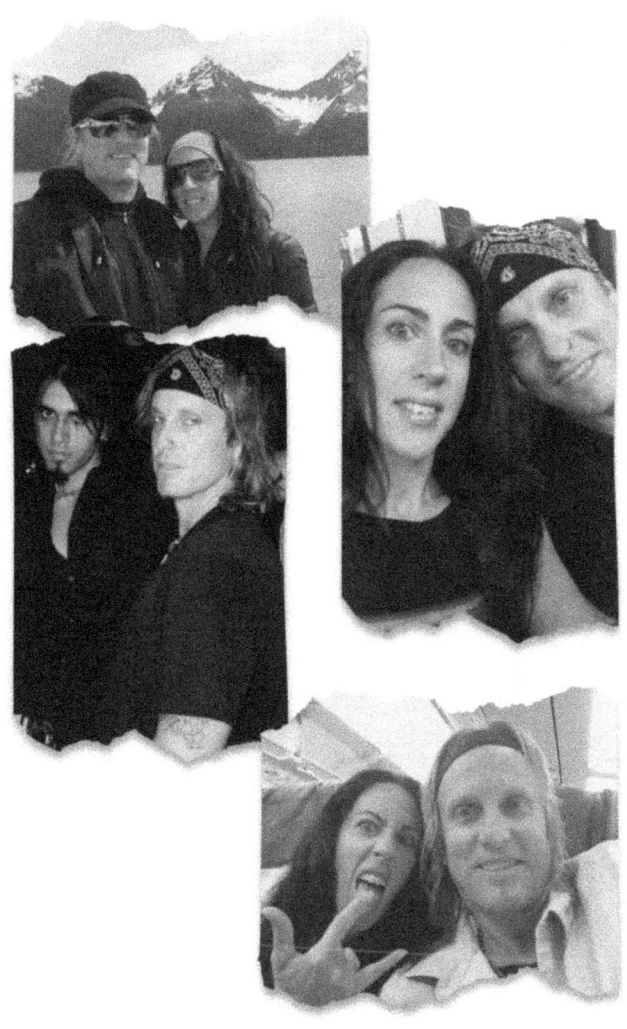

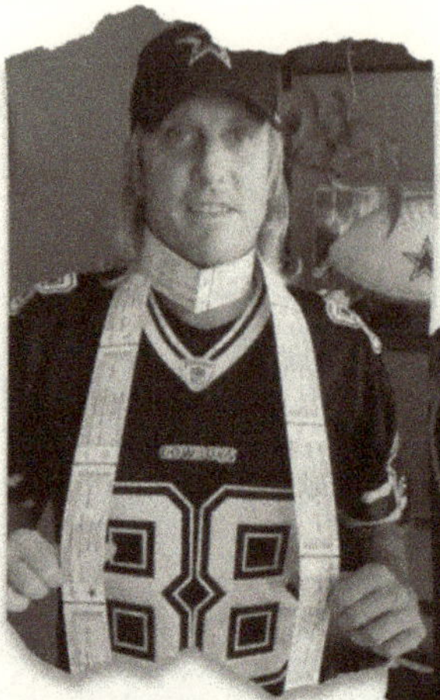

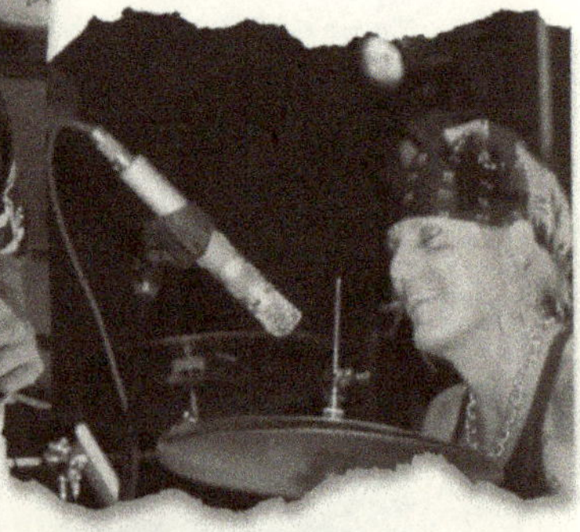

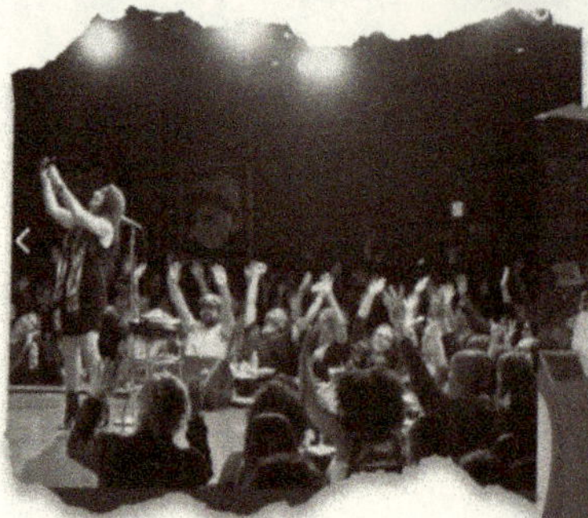

Cali at The Laugh Factory

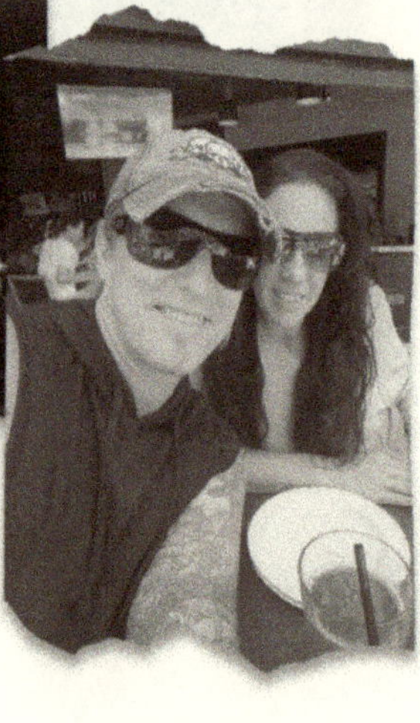

I Married A Junkie – The Final Chapter

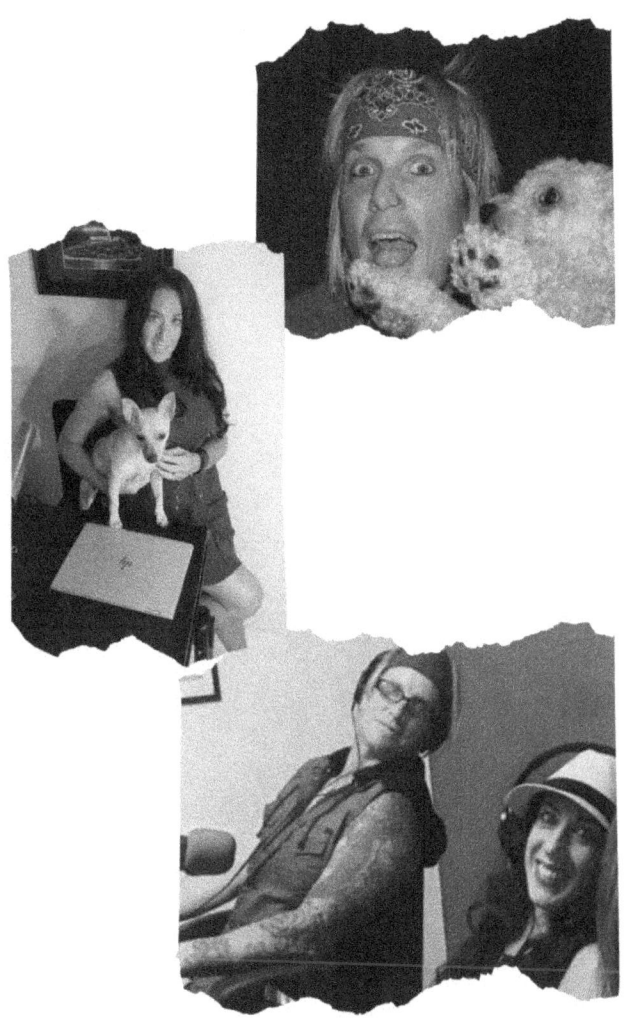

12
Tim

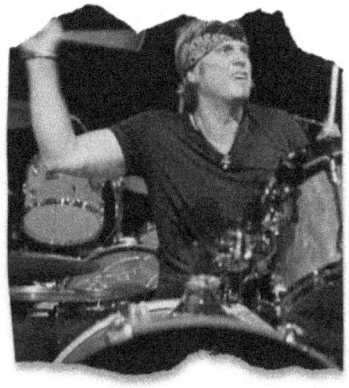

Cali had just bought a Ford F-250 diesel pickup truck in midnight black with matching interior. I was looking forward to getting back on track and starting my own company called All Estes Electric, teaching my son a trade as he moved back from Colorado.

I managed to string six months clean together and I was feeling pretty good. We had our business website up and running, business cards printed, and signs made for the brand-new truck.

I was excited about everything getting started, but in usual fashion, I managed to screw things up before we even got off the ground.

The day after we picked up the truck, I was on my way to help a new client wire an electrical shed. With tools in the back, I was about to pick up my son when I swung through a Shell gas station. I grabbed two taquitos and a Monster energy drink, then filled up the truck. About half a mile down the road, I realized I'd done something incredibly stupid - I'd put gasoline in a diesel truck.

Picture this: I'm pulled over on the side of the road, a mile from the gas station, frantically Googling what happens when you put gas in a diesel truck. I was excited about our first client and launching All Estes Electric that I wasn't thinking when I pumped gas into a brand-new diesel pickup - we'd never owned a diesel before.

A quick search revealed I needed to call a company to pump out the gas, dry the tank, and refill it with diesel. Since I hadn't driven far, the engine should be fine.

I thought I could handle this without upsetting Cali - take care of it, get to the client, wire up their shed, collect the check, and she'd never know there was a problem.

Except when I called to find out the cost of this "fancy trick," it was nearly $1,000, and I had to put it on a credit card. There I was, stranded with the wrong fuel, knowing I couldn't drive anywhere without ruining the engine, facing a $1,000 fix, and Cali was counting on that client's check to cover materials for the next job.

I sat there for about an hour, trying to figure out what to do. I called my son for a ride, but he didn't answer - he had a habit of ignoring calls when he didn't feel social.

After 45 minutes of contemplating cheaper solutions, I bit the bullet and called Cali. She was furious, as expected, but gave me the credit card info. I guess she weighed the cost against potentially replacing a brand-new engine, like we'd done with the Scat Pack, when I forgot an oil change.

I felt terrible about using the client's check for the fuel mix-up instead of supplies. Not wanting to face Cali's anger, I thought maybe I could make up for it by securing more business. My sobriety was clearly at risk if I couldn't keep my head above water with work and income.

These kinds of setbacks, when I don't think things through, really impact us. I get it was an honest mistake, but I guess this was about my 200th "honest mistake" with Cali.

Regardless, she eventually got over it, and we ran All Estes Electric for a very short period.

Suggested Listen:
<u>*Circle the Drain by Wage War*</u>

13
Cali

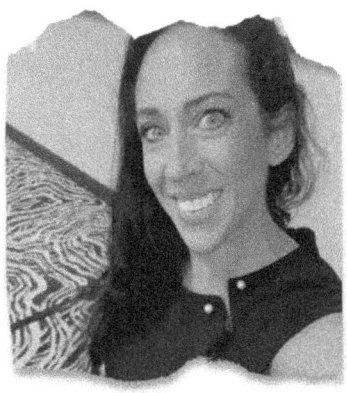

Tim had a short period of sobriety again and things seemed to be mending. We were celebrating my birthday, and I said I wanted to buy an F-350 and deck it out. We went shopping for a new pickup, and I picked out a beautiful white and chrome F-350. I put some rims on it, a lift, and was getting ready to add a Grumper Bumper. I only had it for three days when Tim wrecked it while heavily intoxicated.

He had agreed to go to therapy with me, and we had our first family therapy session with a Gottman therapist.

Gottman therapy is a bit different, focusing on the "Four Horsemen" of unhealthy communication. The therapist we were working with was aware of Tim's addiction and had a strong Alcoholics Anonymous and Big Book orientation.

From the beginning, we explained that Tim wasn't into AA or that type of approach, but it was pushed in the session anyway. Instead of feeling heard and valued, Tim felt attacked and misunderstood. He erupted, feeling like everyone was against him and no one saw his point of view.

Tim grabbed his drums, claiming he was going to rehearsal, even though there wasn't one that night. I told him not to pawn the drums, as they were worth about ten grand. He insisted he was just going to rehearsal, threw the drums in the back of the pickup, and disappeared.

I didn't hear from him for about nine hours, despite calling and texting. No answer.

I had given up at that point. We had a therapy session, but he didn't want to hear what was said or work on things with me. His solution was to obviously go pawn his drums and get high. Addicts have trouble dealing with stress or events where they feel out of control and Tim was no exception.

Around 9:30 that night, I got a call from a cop. I thought it would be that dreaded DOA call, as it wasn't the first time a police officer had called me. The tone in his voice made me believe it was going to be a DOA call, but it wasn't. It was a "come pick up your inebriated husband who just crashed your pickup truck into a pole" call.

I had to track his son down to help me collect the truck and we headed south to get Tim. I decided he was not going to drive any of my vehicles after this. He wrecked every single vehicle we had, except my new wrangler

"Dysel." Every time I set a boundary; Tim steamrolled over it. This time I was going to be firm.

By the time I got there, Tim didn't even know his own name. He was completely out of it, sitting in the front seat in a strange, crouched position. I noticed he wasn't high on the usual substances, but he wasn't himself. The entire front end of my truck was smashed. He had rammed it right into a telephone pole.

I told the cop to arrest him, that I was done and in the process of filing for divorce. The cop said he couldn't arrest Tim because there was no reason - he had only hit a pole, and they had no grounds to arrest him.

I asked if Tim had drugs on him, but the cop said no. I didn't believe it for a second, knowing Tim. He didn't look sober; he didn't look high either.

They released Tim to me. On the way home, he nodded out. The next morning, I asked him what happened. He claimed to have no idea, no memory of how he got there.

The last thing he remembered was buying what he thought was heroin in Fort Pierce, but it turned out to be something else.

Suggested Listen: Save Me by Jelly Roll

14
Tim

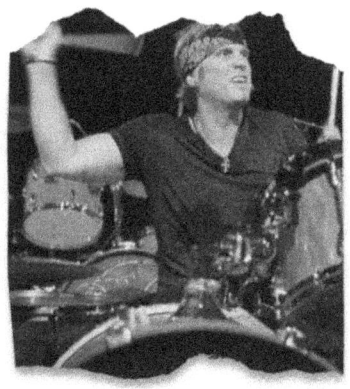

I was doing great, but that old itch to get high was creeping back in. I had a therapy session with Cali. It didn't go well, as always. I always feel like she's accusing me of being a drug addict and not listening to what I'm saying. However, this time I knew I wanted to get high before the session.

I didn't want to do couple's therapy. There was no point. It had taken me years to agree to this, and I had already decided in my head that the minute they brought up AA, I was done. I was out, and I was going to go get high. Cali brought up the topic of divorce and I just didn't want to deal with it.

I ended the session early, figured, "Fuck it." Told Cali I had band rehearsal, grabbed my drums, threw them in the back of the pickup truck to pawn, and went as quickly as I could to a dealer in Fort Pierce that I had met at a gas station the week before while driving the Hellcat. I thought I'd score some heroin. I had never used this guy before. I didn't really know who he was, but I figured I would be just fine, as I always am.

I bought the first bag. It went down easily. The second bag went down easily too. Then I started to feel just a little fuzzy. I thought, "This isn't exactly fentanyl or heroin, but I'm feeling pretty good." I started driving towards Miami. Stopped long enough to pawn my drums and had $1000 to blow.

I don't remember exactly what happened, but it comes in flashes. The first flash was being pulled over at the side of the road after an accident, not sure where. A guy in front of me was screaming at me in Spanish. I must have been in Miami.

I got back in the truck and started driving. Then I thought to myself, "If I just hit somebody, they're looking for me."

I quickly went into Miami to my usual dealer, scored ten bags, put them on my lap and in my mouth around my gums like I normally do, and hightailed it out of there. As I was leaving, I saw cops speeding down into Liberty City, where I just was. They were obviously looking for me.

Heading South, I realized I was going the wrong direction, towards Homestead instead of Hutchinson Island, where we live. I quickly turned around, hoping the cops weren't behind me, trying to stay at the speed limit while sorting bags as I drove. I don't remember anything after that, other than stopping to get a drink because I was thirsty.

The next thing I remember is Cali getting in the truck and yelling at me for crashing the pickup truck. As I think back on the story, flashes of different things come to me.

I think that day the cop asked me to hand him what was in my mouth, and I did. It got me out of trouble because he said if I gave it to him, I could walk. Even when I was high, my mind would work on autopilot, most of the time.

The next day, a cop came to the door to tell me there was a hit and run on the pickup truck. But as usual, I got out of it with a chat with the officer. Told him I was nowhere near the scene.

One of these days, my addiction is going to catch up with me.

Suggested Listen: <u>Live Wire by Mötley Crüe</u>

15
Cali

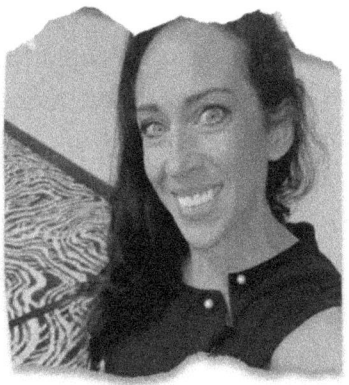

I woke up around 9:15 that morning, still a little groggy, and came out to greet my new puppy, Fozzy, who had been in the house less than a week. I was so excited to have a little puppy because Tim, my husband, had taken to sleeping in a separate room as we were working on a separation towards divorce. He had the two other dogs that would sleep with him.

I drove 12 hours one way to get the puppy, and another 12 hours back. I was excited to see him and walked in to pet him.

That morning, I wasn't prepared for what happened next. Fozzy took about three steps towards me and started to high-pitch whine like he was in severe pain. I tried to pick him up, but he was limp like a rag. He took two more steps, defecated on the floor, and collapsed.

I was screaming for Tim, who was outside. I came running out holding Fozzy, screaming, "We have to get to the vet! We need to get to the emergency vet!"

I didn't even have shoes on or a sweatshirt. We got in the car and drove as quickly as we could to the vet.

Tim was blowing in Fozzy's face, trying to keep him awake. Fozzy kept going limp and unresponsive. I was scared to death something was wrong.

We got to the vet and walked in with an emergency. They took Fozzy to the back and put us in a room. As we were talking, I said to Tim, "I hope he didn't get into your stash."

He insisted he wasn't using and there were no drugs in the house. I made it clear this couldn't happen, as Fozzy was my baby. Tim started yelling, trying to suggest it was my fault, that maybe Fozzy got into my sugar-free gum or plant food for my fruit trees.

The doctor walked in and asked pointedly, "What did he get into?" I had no idea.

The doctor then asked, "What's blue?"

On the top of Fozzy's gum was a blue capsule. Tim claimed to have no idea what it was, but I could see in his eyes he knew.

The doctor noted Tim's pinpoint pupils and asked if he was using opiates. Tim denied it. I was asked who had opiates in the house.

I assured him that there was none that I knew of and explained what I did for a living. I asked if it could be fentanyl. The doctor explained it looked like an opiate overdose and they needed to call poison control.

I Married A Junkie – The Final Chapter

I was panicking, thinking I might lose my dog to an overdose in my own house. I told Tim he needed to come clean about what he was taking.

He continued to deny everything and blame me. I told him I was done, that I wanted a divorce. If this was opiates, I wanted him out of the house, period.

They had to give Fozzy three shots of Narcan. They kept him all day while I waited on pins and needles, worried about the consequences of Tim's reckless drug use.

I was able to pick Fozzy up that night and monitor him, but the incident caused him lasting issues with vision and object permanence.

Tim swore Fozzy had gotten into an old work bag he'd brought in the house years ago and left out by mistake. He promised me he would never touch drugs again, that he was upset by what happened. He had a couple months clean at that point.

I learned several things that day. Tim was no longer using heroin, he was microdosing fentanyl. And once he dumped it all out, he was about to ride the worst detox of his life.

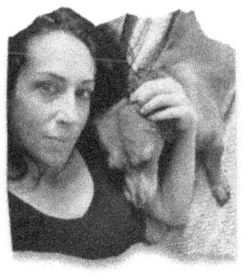

Suggested Listen: <u>Hollywood Hound by CrowFly</u>

You got what you need,
So give me the key
You've been dishonest along the ride
You hit the line

You tripped the line,
And now you can watch it all go by.
Well you better not do it all,
But if you do, don't be afraid

So get up
Get up and take your day,
I'm taking back my way,
Learning to read the signs,
So come on, come on
You had better heed your pace,
There ain't no time to waste
Killing time was all I ever, all I ever was.

You're losing your mind,
You're losing control,
You know you've lost it all
A thousand times.

You hit the wall,
You built it strong

I Married A Junkie – The Final Chapter

And now you can watch
It all go by.

So get up
Get up and take your day,
I'm taking back my way,
Learning to read the signs,
So come on, come on
You had better heed your pace,
There ain't no time to waste
Killing time was all I ever, all I ever was.

Killing time was all I ever was,
All I ever was, it's all I ever was.

Songwriters: Brandon James and Tim Estes

Lyrics © Brandon James and Tim Estes

16
Cali

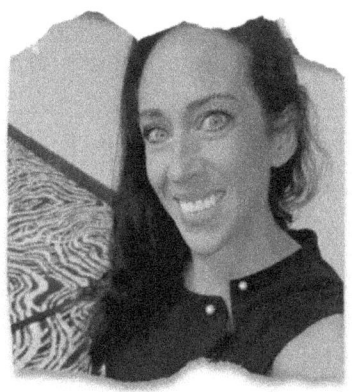

Tim's son had lived in Colorado for a few years. We had bought him a car and set him up in a townhouse there so he could be near his brother and build a career. When he couldn't sustain himself, he called to come back. We decided to let him stay in our RV at the park, where he and Tim would start All Estes Electric, teaching Tim's son a trade. This seemed like the best solution at the time.

I reluctantly agreed to let him stay in the RV because of how he'd left the Colorado house.

I had to fly out and fix damages that were left behind to prep the house for sale. With Tim out of commission, it was one more big project that fell into my lap. Trying to run a company, a household and parent an adult child was too much to do alone. I was hoping all my hard work would pay off and Tim could get sober permanently and step up as a husband and a father.

They started All Estes Electric and got a few clients. The plan was for me to fund the promotional materials, marketing, and website to get them started, and they'd pay me back.

Over the next year, they had to go back to regular jobs because they couldn't get the company off the ground or pay for supplies. Tim kept charging my credit card for supplies and using job payments to buy drugs. I told him I was done and wouldn't continue at this pace.

Then COVID hit, causing panic. I immediately moved us out of Miami, we had a condo and lived on the 40th floor in Brickell. The condo complex shut down the pool, the gym and the elevator. That meant walking two dogs up and down 40 flights of stairs, in the heat, three times a day. I couldn't do it, not to mention there were no gyms open.

We moved up to a rental house in Boynton Beach. It was near the RV park where his son was living. We ended up having severe black mold issues in that rental almost immediately. Of course, the landlords were not willing to fix it, and nothing was open, it was awful for me as I am highly allergic to mold.

I was over landlords at this point, and the housing market was going up. I decided that we should buy a house and get some investment real estate once again.

We ended up buying a house on Hutchinson Island - my first home purchase for us to reside in, which should have been a wonderful experience. Unfortunately, things went south quickly.

Tim and I were desperately trying to work on our marriage. His idea was to get a house with a mother-in-law suite so his son could stay there for six months, start working, save money, and then get his own apartment.

I reluctantly agreed, despite having already bought him a house in Colorado and two vehicles. But Tim always got his way. We agreed to six months only so we could rent out the extra apartment on this property.

When I went to clean up the RV to sell or move it, I was horrified. His son hadn't taken care of it at all, and it was left to me once again to handle.

I had another long talk with both about mutual respect, working, and contributing. Everyone agreed to pitch in with this new house, keep it clean and work on upgrading it. I was mentally and physically exhausted. I couldn't keep doing this with them. I needed a partner, and I wanted the old Tim back.

Tim had been clean for four months. He was prone to chronic relapse - he'd get clean, do well for a while, then relapse.

He couldn't get out of his own way, and everything triggered him: stress, his son's inability to be an adult in his mid-twenties, feeling his band was falling apart due to COVID. He'd often say, "I don't know who I am anymore" because he wasn't playing music.

His attempts to connect with his other son would fall flat as well. He seemed lost.

All these factors drove him to use, but he'd pull himself out with his recovery coach, therapist, or sober companion, getting back on track temporarily. Tim had access to the best care through my company, Sober on Demand, with top sober companions, therapists, and coaches. He'd do great for a while, then something would happen, and he would spiral down again. This became his norm.

When sober, I'd catch glimpses of the wonderful person I first met. He'd give you the shirt off his back, give his last dollar to a homeless person, and talk with them for hours. He was truly an amazing human being.

But drugs ravaged him and his brain. As he moved from heroin to microdosing fentanyl, which has a horrible detox, he became a shell of his former self. I spared no expense trying to help him, from detoxes to live-in sober companions, but the cycle continued.

Suggested Listen: Surrender by Godsmack

17
Cali

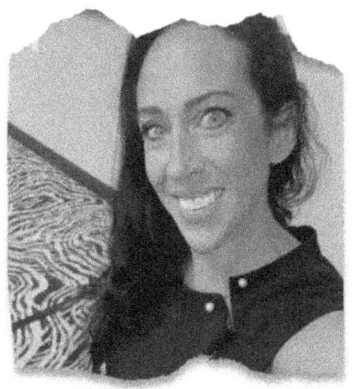

Buying a house for the first time is a huge milestone, but purchasing a -million-dollar beach house is an even bigger deal. Doing it without a partner contributing financially, while also supporting his nearly 30-year-old son who refused to work, made it a monumental challenge.

The house we bought on Hutchinson Island was a sprawling three-bedroom, six-bath home with a separate mother-in-law suite. It boasted the largest pool on the island, a hot tub, an additional outdoor bath, and spanned two lots.

The house was enormous, and so was the mortgage payment. But I was excited that it could be used for my Sober on Demand private clients since it was beachside and could be used as an Airbnb. We closed on the house during the COVID pandemic and Tim had almost 8 months clean.

I was thrilled to sign the papers after all the hard work it took to secure the loan and get everything in order. We put the house in both our names, although I was the primary borrower.

To celebrate, we picked up some ahi sandwiches from Manatee Grill, planning to eat in the new house and toast to a fresh start and better life. I was happy, I thought for sure being almost two hours from Miami would ground him and he could surf and help me run the Airbnb.

We arrived at the house and let the dogs out back. We hadn't even been there a minute, admiring the beautiful yard, when I turned to tell Tim how happy I was that he was sober, and we were getting back on track.

That's when I saw he had nodded out and crumpled to the ground. I went over to check on him and saw his eyes rolled back in his head. He had gotten high again, for the umpteenth time, in a moment that meant so much to me. I had worked hard to get here and just wanted to celebrate briefly, but he chose drugs instead.

After his eyes rolled back, I managed to get him inside and laid him down in the Florida room. He was breathing and moaning slightly, but I was utterly done. I wanted a divorce. I knew right then that I was finished with him.

For the past decade, he had ruined every positive event and everything I had tried to build with him as a team. He had thrown it all away to yet again cheat on me with opiates. It broke my heart. This was a dream of mine to own a beach house and have a sober service right onsite.

When active addicts want to use, they don't care about anyone but themselves. I knew this in my heart and mind. At this point, I felt I was enabling him. I left him on the floor, took the dogs, and drove back to our rental unit an hour away.

About two hours later, he called asking where I was. I told him it should have been one of the happiest days of my life, but it was miserable because he couldn't stay sober.

Of course, he lied and tried to say he wasn't high. I told him I had watched him lying on the floor for nearly an hour, making sure he was breathing and wouldn't die, before I left. I told him I wanted a divorce.

This wasn't the first time I had asked for a divorce, more like the tenth. He would never agree to it. He always wanted half of everything plus alimony, and after consulting several attorneys, I learned he was entitled to it.

Not only would he get half of everything I had built, but also 40% of my income for life. He likely wouldn't make it that long, with the quantity of drugs he was using and the money he was blowing on gambling, fancy cars, and whatever else he wanted. He would probably be busted and destitute, if not dead from an overdose, within six months.

I told him I couldn't do it anymore and hung up. The next day, I called a realtor and said I wanted to put the house on the market, even though I had just closed on it. I didn't want to live there. She informed me that in Florida, I would have to wait a year to sell it due to tax and property rights issues. I was stuck in this for another year.

We ended up moving into the house on Christmas Eve. He laid in bed, complaining we were making too much noise as we unpacked.

There were no presents on Christmas Day; there hadn't been for years, at least not for me. I always made sure he and his child had a good Christmas, but they never really remembered me.

Suggested Listen: <u>High on Me by Saliva</u>

18
Tim

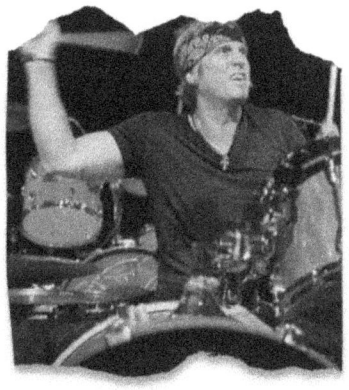

Cali told me she was done. I vowed to try to win her back and keep her, and my son and I started working on the house. I detoxed myself off Fentanyl yet again and headed to Home Depot for supplies to redo the bathrooms.

The day in reference started out like any other normal day. I noticed a lady frantically waving her arms trying to get someone to pull over and help her. No one was stopping, and I pulled over to help. I saw a dog in the grass by the side of the road, and it couldn't use its back legs.

"Oh my god a car just hit my dog!" she yelled.

I got out, lifted the dog and took her and the lady to the hospital right around the corner.

After an hour inside the pet emergency room, the vet informed us that the dog, Tinkerbell, had a broken pelvis and would need to go to the local pet surgeon immediately to get her pelvis repaired. The dog was likely in a lot of pain and would need pain meds for the ride.

Now this is the kind of thing that a drug addict like me usually wants to hear. Pain meds on tap!!!! Except I am a huge dog lover and would not put the dog in jeopardy. We gave the dog pain meds, and I drove the lady and her dog to the surgeon.

The vet gave us the $400 vet bill and the lady began to cry. She didn't have the $400, but since I still had Cali's credit card from the store, I paid for it. This would be my good deed for the week.

Once we got the dog to the surgeon's office an hour from home, Stuart Animal Hospital claimed the dog was worse off than just a broken pelvis and told us that if we didn't give them $4,000, they were going to refuse the dog into care.

We told them not to treat the dog and wanted her put back into the truck and we would go elsewhere.

They refused. In fact, they demanded $4000. I called Cali and got a green light to pay for it. But I was livid. I called the surgeon out, "I either give you $4,000 or you let this dog die?!"

I love animals, there is no way I am going to let this dog die even though this vet surgeon is acting totally unethically. I decided to deal with that later and focus on saving the poor dog's life. A dog that wasn't even mine.

After two days, the surgeon called to inform me that the dog had lived and was doing much better. However, they claimed to have spent the entire $4,000 "saving the dog's life with oxygen and pain meds" and now needed another $4,000 to do the pelvic surgery.

I paid $4000 for the surgery, and they did not even do it! The vet sent her home with a prescription of Hydrocodone in hopes that the dog's owner would come up with another $4,000 for the surgery.

This is where even more unbelievable chaos began. Remember I said getting pain meds on tap was an addict's dream? Yeah, here we go.

I thought I won the lotto with this prescription, except, pharmacy after pharmacy kept refusing to fill the pain pill prescription.

They didn't care how bad the dog was in pain, they didn't want to talk to the vet, and one after another kept refusing to fill the prescription. The dog had a broken pelvis and was in severe pain. I was not going to let this happen.

I called my old drug dealer in Miami and went down to pick up some hydrocodone.

I should have called Cali and had her help me find a pharmacy, but I figured my brilliant plan was better. And as we know, all my plans turn out brilliantly.

I made it to Miami and grabbed the dog's meds and a few extra 'just in case.'

I told myself I wouldn't do them, but by the time I was back to the lady's house I had snorted those and dipped into the dog's stash. Twenty-four hours later and I was back to microdosing fentanyl.

My plan was brilliant, until it wasn't.

Suggested Listen: <u>Psycho by Asking Alexandria</u>

19
Cali

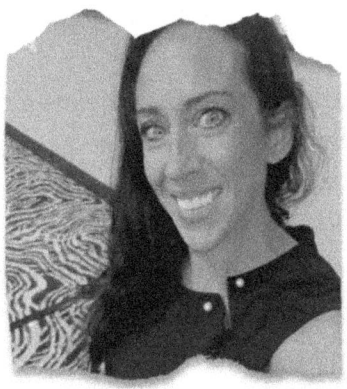

I certainly wasn't expecting Homeland Security to show up at my house, at least not this way. We had barely been in our new home for a few months when I was jolted awake by a thud.

The sound was everything on my kitchen counter falling off as Tim slid sideways, holding onto the counter before cracking his head on the floor. He was overdosing, turning blue and foaming at the mouth.

I shot out of bed, called 911, and quickly corralled the dogs in their crates. I don't even remember what I said to the operator. They kept asking seemingly irrelevant questions, and all I could say was, "He's turning blue. You need to get here now."

Within minutes, four cop cars, an ambulance, and Homeland Security arrived. All told, there were eleven officers (three from Homeland Security), and four EMTs in my house.

They administered Narcan, requiring three doses as usual, before loading Tim into the ambulance and taking him to the hospital.

Meanwhile, I had to deal with eleven officers in my living room, asking me countless questions. When I asked what they were looking for, Homeland Security said they were searching for any illegal aliens I might be harboring - a bizarre situation given we'd just moved in, and I called 911 to report a drug interaction/poisoning.

After about 45 minutes, I finally convinced them to leave as they found no drug paraphernalia. They asked me to come to the station for questioning, which I refused after asking, "Am I being detained?" They said no.

Having worked with high-profile clients who've had legal troubles, I've learned to always ask if I'm being detained. If not, politely decline. If arrested, say nothing and ask for a lawyer.

Apparently, we were the youngest people on the block and had the largest piece of property beachside, we were seen as suspicious at the jump.

This experience left a bad taste in my mouth regarding how people treat addicts and their families. I didn't appreciate how the police treated us like criminals.

The lead officer, the only woman in the group, kept pressing me for his dealer's phone number. I didn't know who his dealer was, what he took, or where he got it. We'd barely been in the area, and I didn't have any answers to her questions.

I Married A Junkie – The Final Chapter

She wasn't happy with him (and me either) and they were scouring my house looking for any paraphernalia.

They found nothing.

I followed the ambulance to the hospital but had to wait three to four hours before they released him. This was a new process they claimed they had to follow once Narcan was used.

By the time they released him, he was stone cold sober and furious at me.

Narcan is a mix of Naloxone and Buprenorphine, it cleans your system out once you take it and that means that your high is completely gone and you are sober.

It also poses another issue, the medical staff never seem to inform their patients that once they administer Narcan, their body will not need or tolerate the same amount of the drugs they used to use to get high. This means their tolerance level declines.

Most addicts will go right back to using the same amount they took right before they got the Narcan. This will cause an overdose and death. A lot of overdoses can be avoided with this simple communication at the hospital or from the EMT's.

What struck me most was how the hospital staff treated him - not as a person in need, but as trash. Instead of asking if he was okay, needed therapy, or was having mental health issues, they treated him like a problem clogging up the ER.

I also noticed others in the ER suffering from mental illness being treated similarly.

He would end up at Lawnwood Hospital again, when his artery burst and the ER doctor would stall service, because he called him a 'junkie' that was probably drinking too much and 'going to die anyway.'

He was bleeding to death and would end up intubated in the ICU.

This horrendous experience prompted me to create a class on mental health addiction coaching to help others in this situation. I also developed first responder training to teach police, doctors and EMT's how to deal with mental health and addiction cases.

No family should ever feel like a problem or burden when calling for help. First responders should reassure families that their loved ones will be okay, not make them feel uncomfortable or criminalized.

As you've seen in both books, there's a theme in how people with addiction are treated - as less than or unworthy. This shouldn't be the case.

I hope these books bring awareness to mental health issues and drug addiction, offering solutions and proper training.

This is why I founded The Addictions Academy and our partner company, Addiction and Mental Health Training, found at AAMHT.com, the largest provider of online, webinar, in-person, and self-study addiction and mental health classes globally. We offer comprehensive courses on addiction, mental health, trauma, and various types of addiction.

I created this because of how my husband was treated for so long. I had realized there's not enough training for people to help others effectively and humanely.

Suggested Listen:
Don't Tell Me by Disturbed and Ann Wilson

20
Tim

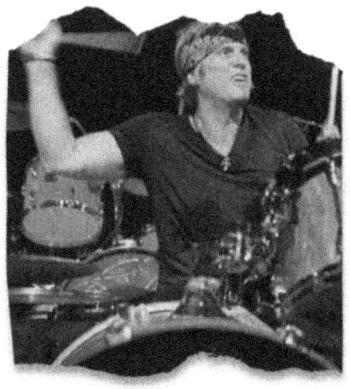

I'm a very private person when it comes to deaths in my immediate family and my own medical issues. I don't need or want the attention that comes with these situations. On August 28, 2022, my life took an unexpected turn.

I stood up in my living room, and the next thing I remember, my wife was screaming. I found myself face-first on the floor, blood everywhere from a head wound.

What I didn't know then was that a very sharp gallstone had cut an artery between my liver and gallbladder. I had been bleeding internally for about 8 days without realizing it.

I had an aneurysm and was completely unaware.

I passed out because the slow internal bleeding had caused my oxygen level to drop as low as 58% (normal is 98-99%).

The hospital was more concerned with stitching up my forehead than addressing my breathing difficulties. They yelled at me to stop pulling away as they stitched my head.

When they finally realized my dangerously low oxygen levels, they placed a child-sized oxygen mask over my mouth - it was all they could find. It didn't fit, it didn't work, and I lost consciousness.

The next thing I remember is waking up in the ICU with a tube down my throat. The doctor informed me about my aneurysm and that my gallbladder was "full" of razor-sharp stones that needed removal immediately. I had been given 15 pints of blood and would be in the ICU for five days.

They gave me pain medication every four hours - 10mg Roxies. Just what an ex-heroin addict needs, right? After three days, the Roxies stopped working, and they switched to liquid Dilaudid directly into my IV. This continued for another four days. By day eight, my brain receptors were hooked on opiates once again.

On Day 1 in the emergency room, after they intubated me, the doctor told my wife, right in front of my son, to pre-sign my death paperwork because I had less than a 1% chance of surviving surgery. The ICU doctor mistakenly thought I had brain damage from the fall.

On Day 8, they informed me they couldn't give me any more painkillers and needed to sedate me for a throat camera procedure. I explained that to stop the opiates cold turkey would cause withdrawals, but they dismissed my concerns.

Fed up with their lack of understanding, I stood up, removed my own IV and monitors, got dressed, and walked out the front door against medical advice. The staff followed me to the elevator, warning me I would die.

You can probably guess where I went next - straight to Liberty City to get some fentanyl caps. I didn't want to get sick, and the thought of vomiting and ripping my stitches was too much. My "brilliant" plan was to score about 30 caps and wean myself off once I healed properly. But we all know how well my brilliant plans go.

Two weeks later, I was once again fully addicted, telling myself I could stop whenever I wanted - I was just "healing."

Suggested Listen:
Let's Get the Party Started by Tom Morello and Bring Me the Horizon

21
Tim

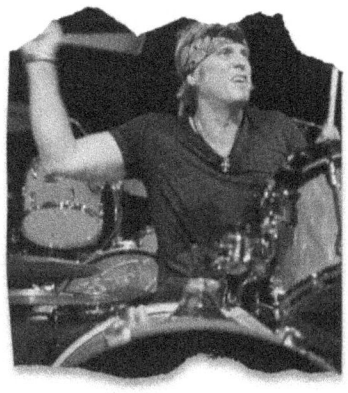

Microdosing is a funny word, and its meaning is interpreted differently from user to user. I've always microdosed cocaine a bit to keep the heroin or fentanyl urges at bay after the physical withdrawals are over.

I don't recommend this for others, but it always worked for me. Except the final time during the final detox. This one is a little more horrifying than entertaining, so buckle up!

With pills and heroin detoxes, I always seemed to snap back into shape after two weeks. With this latest fentanyl detox, I'm on Day 14, and psychologically, I feel no better than Day 5.

I'm realizing that this fentanyl withdrawal is a whole different animal. Remember my minor adjustments? Here's my final one.

Microdosing cocaine during the later stages of detox has always worked for me, so let's do it again. I have always been able to put cocaine down, and it is not physical with me. It's all psychological.

Let me rephrase that. When I was young and broke, I really struggled with putting coke down. But later in life, when I could afford as much coke as I could snort, it became a take-it-or-leave-it thing for me. But you never know when old demons may reappear when actively using drugs.

Obviously, I scored some powder and began to "microdose" cocaine to feel better. How fucked up does that sound?

I purchased eight high tops. High tops in Miami are twenty-dollar bags, or pillows, as my band used to call them.

I'm going to "microdose" these eight bags of cocaine for eight days. Remember, all my drug-induced plans are perfect, and this one is no exception. A twenty-dollar bag of coke is enough to keep my fentanyl urges at bay but not enough to set me back. I'm good.

Here we are, fourteen days removed from a cold turkey fentanyl detox and about five months removed from a cystic artery aneurysm that almost killed me.

Let me explain this cystic artery aneurysm again. There are only twenty-seven known cases of people who have had the type of aneurysm I had. Well, twenty-eight now. And many of those cases were pseudo-aneurysms. This means, in those cases, the artery never burst or ruptured.

Mine ruptured, and I slowly bled for eight days until I face-planted my tile floor and was rushed to the hospital. Here's where my addictive mind got sickening.

The first bag of coke went flawlessly. It always does. I had energy, no fentanyl urges, I was focused and feeling creative as hell for the first time in a long time. This shit is magic! If I feel this good from one bag, imagine how I'll feel if I open a second.

Now two key bumps into the second bag, I feel a slight spasm in the middle of my abdomen right below my ribs. Now, this is close to where my aneurysm was.

This is where I start bargaining with my addictive mind. I remember that my phone has all the answers, and I Google my spasm symptoms. And I'm high on coke.

Google tells me that it's probably a diaphragm spasm and nothing to worry about, but it could be the sign of a heart attack, stroke, or aneurysm.

I decided it's just a diaphragm spasm and do another bump of coke, compliments of my addictive mind. I totally dismiss the other serious possibilities that can be brought on by cocaine use.

A few minutes later, I just didn't feel right.

After you go from microdosing cocaine to abusing it, paranoia will always set in. This will come into full play for the rest of the first night. Not feeling right, I get up to use the restroom, and as I'm relieving myself, I happen to look in the mirror.

My face looked like I had been at the beach all day. And I haven't been in the sun for almost a decade because of opiates. I decided it's my blood pressure, and I have a great blood pressure machine that I bought when I walked out of the hospital. I checked my blood pressure daily after the aneurysm, let's see what's going on.

I put the cuff on, high on coke, upside down, and hit go.

I have no idea if you have ever put a blood pressure cuff upside down but if not, here's what happens. Just having the cuff upside down will cause a much higher reading. Couple that with cocaine, and your reading will be ridiculous.

My first reading came back 148/111. Fuck! I'm about to die! I tell myself that the spasm was the artery, my red face is from ridiculous blood pressure, and I'm about to stroke out.

How quickly microdosing has turned into certain death, and my awesome feeling has turned into sheer terror. I close my eyes and wait for my impending stroke.

Thirty minutes later, I felt better. I was just paranoid. At least I think so. But let's take my blood pressure again just to be safe.

That's when I realized that I put the cuff upside down and I reassured myself I would be fine, like I always am.

Suggested Listen: *Pray for Me by Sixx: A.M.*

22
Cali

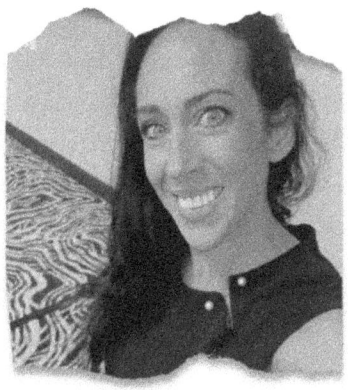

The day Tim died started like any other. He had 29 days clean from microdosing fentanyl and, as I learned that day, from speedballing on and off for nearly a decade.

By speedballing, I mean he was combining opiates with either crack cocaine or powder cocaine to "get his mind right."

When clients first come off heavy opiates, the initial days are primarily physical - sleeping a lot, vomiting, diarrhea, restless legs, sweats, and nausea. Then they start to feel better physically and begin eating, but that's when the mental challenges set in.

First comes anger. They're furious, often directing it at those closest to them. They're angry about having to quit. Their brain's neuroreceptors aren't firing properly, manifesting as rage.

Then comes the victim mentality - crying, sadness, even suicidal thoughts. This is typically when they might relapse or use stimulants to boost their neurotransmitters.

On this day, Tim was cycling through all these emotions. He was angry because he wanted Dunkin' Donuts, but I reminded him he'd had major surgery six months ago and was supposed to be eating healthy. Our deal was always that if he wanted junk food, he wouldn't eat it at home.

What I didn't know until after he passed was the extent of his junk food addiction - pizza, taquitos, 7-11 food, fast food, donuts, energy drinks, sugar. His diet was awful, but he did honor me by not bringing it into the house.

That day, when I told him to eat healthily, he started screaming and throwing things. Just another day in a typical detox cycle.

I had Suboxone on hand to lessen his symptoms, yet he refused to take it. He said he was going to visit a friend across the state. Before leaving, he suggested we have sushi. Then Tim, his son, and I went out for what would be my last meal with him.

During the meal, I tried to discuss the upcoming Airbnb rental and his son moving out, but Tim interjected, saying he wanted to talk about the Dallas Cowboys instead.

His detox-induced anger and fits of rage made me feel like nothing mattered. I was done, realizing the situation wasn't going to improve if he continued using and detoxing in an endless loop.

I Married A Junkie – The Final Chapter

The original plan for this property was to split the main house in two sections and rent both out along with the mother-in-law suite that his son was still living in. We were even in the process of getting permits for two tiny homes to add to the income on the property.

About four hours later, he loaded the pickup and headed to his friend's place. He called on the way, still combative and argumentative.

I told him I was done. I just couldn't deal with this anymore and I reiterated my desire for divorce, and finally, he agreed to sign the paperwork.

Previously, he'd only agree if I gave him half of everything, which would have been disastrous given his addictions, but now I was just exhausted.

I couldn't carry the company, him, his kid, and all the bills that went along with this massive house that just kept going up. My monthly payment doubled in less than a year. I couldn't get the financial support from Tim, or his son to move out, allowing me to rent the place which was the original plan.

I was exhausted from months of caretaking - being at his ICU bedside for 12 hours a day for eight days, running my company, caring for multiple dogs (including his son's unfriendly Pit bull-Doberman mix), managing all the household issues, while his family offered little to no support. His brother, living just an hour away, never visited during Tim's hospital stay or recovery.

During our last phone conversation, Tim seemed off. When I asked if he was okay, he insisted he was fine and again agreed to sign the divorce papers upon his return.

I immediately printed out the divorce paperwork and the house sale contract, placing them on the counter.

After walking the dogs and getting ready for bed, I texted him to ensure he was okay. He mentioned he stopped by McDonald's and got a double cheeseburger, fries and a coke.

I told him that was probably not a good idea as he was clean from fast food and sugar for six months. And his system probably couldn't handle that with his gallstones. He said he would be fine, and he would call me tomorrow.

I went to bed.

I never saw or spoke to him again after that.

Suggested Listen: Over and Over by CrowFly

Pause your speech for just a moment
Place your eyes on me.
Let's take a minute and reflect
 This cold heart, tragic.

What are lies
When you believe anything that shadows me.
But I carried all of your weight
And pretend we are so happy.

Over and over
I had to wait
I never meant to walk away
But you never meant to stay.

Over and over
I felt this way
I never meant to walk away
But you never meant to stay.

Looking back it's so surreal
How I fell for all your tears,
Such a rotting heart
And a pretty face to hide it.

What are lies
When you believe anything that shadows me.
But I carried all of your weight
And pretend we are so happy.

Over and over
I had to wait
I never meant to walk away
But you never meant to stay

Over and over
I felt this way
I never meant to walk away
But you never meant to stay.

All my words are blind,
heed your precious time
Keep my pain inside
Bring me to my knees

But I was alive,
I was alive.
But I carried all of your weight
And pretend we are so happy.

Over and over
I had to wait
I never meant to walk away
But you never meant to stay

Over and over
I felt this way
Over and over
I had to wait
I never meant to walk away
But you never meant to stay

Over and over
I felt this way,
All my words are blind,
Heed your precious time
Keep my pain inside

Want me to pretend...
I won't.

Songwriters: Brandon James and Tim Estes

Lyrics © Brandon James and Tim Estes

23
Cali

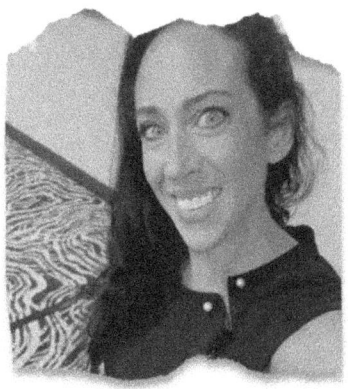

The call came the next morning from Tim's friend. He asked if I had heard from Tim, and I said no. I had texted him a few times to check in but received no response.

The friend said Tim's bedroom door was locked, and he couldn't get in.

At that moment, I knew something was very wrong.

The night before, Tim had butt dialed me at 9:14 pm and it sounded like his phone was in his pocket. I said "hello, hello" but no response. I hung up.

He dialed back at 9:15 pm and same thing. This was not odd, as Tim would keep his phone in his pocket and butt dial me all the time.

But this time I had an odd feeling, like something was not right. I called him back and there was no answer.

I have had odd feelings before, and of course being married to an active drug user there is always a sense of panic when you cannot reach your partner.

I told myself, I was being paranoid, he was feeling better when he left, we had just spoken, and all was well.

Except it wasn't.

I told Tim's friend to break down the door.

He did. I heard him scream and drop the phone. When he picked it up again, he told me Tim was dead.

I asked him to describe the scene. He said Tim was at the end of his bed, on his knees with his head back, and there was vomit all over the floor. It looked like he had stood up to go to the bathroom, vomited, and then couldn't get back up.

After the police arrived, I asked if they found any drugs around him or signs of drug use. They said no.

Later, I learned that he had probably had a heart attack and re-injured the aneurysm, causing it to burst, along with his heart at the same time.

The doctor explained that the stress of the day, the detox, cocaine use in the past few days, the four-hour drive, and stopping for a cheeseburger, fries, and a large Coca-Cola likely pushed his body into overdrive, triggering the heart attack.

His death certificate reads "natural causes, heart attack."

His body simply gave out.

I wasn't entirely surprised. Tim was a long-term drug user who always promised that he would quit opiates for good.

We met when he was 38 and did not use heavily. He'd drink occasionally, nothing extreme, same with his cocaine use. But when he found opiates in his mid-forties, he couldn't put them down.

He'd always say, "I'm stopping at 45... 46... 47... 48." When he turned 50, he swore he'd be done. But it never happened.

Instead, his use seemed to escalate. Once he started opiates, he couldn't stop. He would always say that it kept the demons at bay.

I knew he felt guilty for not being a great dad to the son living with us and awful for not having a relationship with his other son.

Heroin and Fentanyl made the chatter in his brain just go away and everything seemed like roses. He made me listen to the song 'Heroin' by Badflower once, and he said, "This is what getting high on heroin feels like."

Here I was, taking this call outside, realizing the dogs are barking, there was food on the stove, and I had work to do... immediate, time-pressing work. I was in the process of coordinating a client and a sober companion, making phone calls and running my business. How was I supposed to process this?

An hour later, my staff pitched in to cover for me and I was on the road with Tim's son to pick up the truck and Tim's suitcase from across the state.

The 3 ½ hour drive felt like 10 hours. I texted Tim's mother and brothers and got no response.

About 2 hours into the drive, I got a call from his cousin, asking what was going on and I told him. He told me that the family thought I was joking about Tim's death, and they had been calling him, but his phone was dead.

Mind you, the family never called me or texted me, and who jokes about death?

Next thing I know his cousin called a friend and WHAM!

The phone was ringing off the hook, Facebook posts everywhere. One of Tim's old friends from high school even posted that "her first love had passed away."

FUCK!!!

I couldn't even get a minute to wrap my head around it and everyone he knew was calling. And Tim knew A LOT of people.

Most of the calls were the standard question "what happened?" Not if I was OK or needed anything – and I hadn't even posted he passed on Facebook yet.

In the midst of all this, one of Tim's good friends, Kimmi Jones called, and she literally stopped the madness. She took care of the calls among Tim's high school friends and gave me room to breathe.

Tim's cousin owned a funeral home and offered to handle the cremation and funeral/celebration of life arrangements. However, I chose not to hold a funeral or a celebration of life. I wasn't ready to celebrate someone who had caused me so much pain in recent years.

I didn't want to listen to everyone share amazing stories when I had been living in hell for so long.

Moreover, the family would expect me to organize and pay for the whole thing.

In hindsight, maybe I should have held that celebration of life. What was to come next would prove far more painful than what had just happened.

Suggested Listen:
The Death of Peace of Mind by Bad Omens

24
Cali

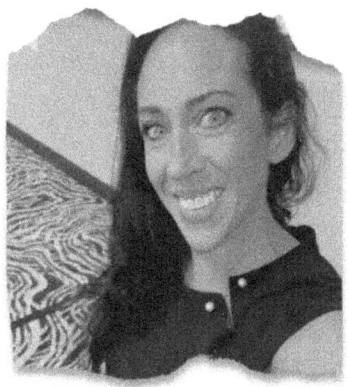

Not only did I not expect to be a widow at 48, I also never expected to have to call the police on my stepson to have him removed from my property.

After multiple calls to the family for help and getting little assistance and a lot of excuses, I had to take action to get his son out of the apartment.

Tim was an amazing entertainer and drummer, but he would never parent. Now I was left to navigate this by myself.

Over the years, Tim's family never visited, they only called when they wanted something financial or help from Tim.

From fixing an AC, house repairs or assorted tasks, his brothers always seemed to be working less and expecting their mother to cover their mortgages, car payments - even gifts for their wives.

I was probably too outspoken, but after I helped them financially repair the pool, bought his mom a new dryer and other appliances, and filled the fridge multiple times, I had to say something when I learned what was really going on. Tim and I discovered that one brother and his wife were basically living there rent free with another brother siphoning his mother's retirement account to pay his rent, car, credit cards, Instacart and even Western Union himself her cash... I was over it.

No one should exploit their mother like that. These were grown men with wives. Why they couldn't work, or more accurately wouldn't work was baffling.

But I knew why.

If you remember in the first ***I Married A Junkie*** book, Tim talked about how his parents gave him everything, and fixed all his problems.

It seemed the same way with both of his brothers, no one could 'adult'. Every issue they had was fixed by mom and dad. And when Tim's dad passed away in 2016, Tim stepped in to fix the problems himself.

He did repair work on his house, and his brother's house. When his brother needed a ride to the hospital for open heart surgery, Tim drove up there and took him to Orlando, waited for him to come out of surgery and stayed with him.

When Tim had his aneurysm burst and went to the ICU, I called his brother, and he was supposed to meet me

at the hospital. He never showed up. Nor did any family members come during the 5 days in ICU or the hospital.
NOT.
ONE.
VISIT.
Why I expected help from them was probably delusional on my part. In fact, their behavior got worse. Death and money clearly tear people apart.

This is how it all went down.

I had a friend over helping me with things at the house, four days after learning of Tims' death (Thank you to Dr. Terri Sell, my ProRecovery RX business partner that jumped in and just handled 'all the things' that needed to be handled).

Suddenly, I noticed a pit bull in my side yard.

I called my stepson who was supposed to be in the apartment clearing it out for an Airbnb renter, and he put me on speaker phone.

I asked him whose dog was in the yard and whose truck was in the driveway. He said he was in his apartment, with his mother.

Yes, the same one that stole the car I gave him when he was 16 so she could buy drugs. The same one that threatened to kill me because I wouldn't give her money, that one. I hadn't seen or spoken to her for 14 years and suddenly she was in my apartment, on my property, with her dog within three days of Tim's passing.

While on the speaker phone, his mom informed me that she has suddenly become homeless and brought all her belongings over.

The expectation seemed to be that because she was suddenly homeless, she would live in the mother-in-law suite with my stepson, with neither of them paying rent or bills while I footed all the expenses of the property.

I wasn't having it. I wasn't going to let my stepson disrespect me that way, let alone his mother who had threatened my life years ago, living in my house rent-free.

She wasn't in his life in the last 14 years that I was feeding him, clothing him, housing him etc. I had bought him three vehicles and a townhouse, several phones, and given him money to start a company.

This is what I ended up with.

But wait, it got worse.

I tried to convince him to move his things out of the apartment. It was Airbnb season, and I needed the extra cash to cover the ridiculous insurance and tax bill that went up to $40,000 per year. Then add the mortgage on top, plus all the utilities, lawn service, pool service, tree service, etc. I felt like I was drowning.

The extra income from the Airbnb rental would cover all those expenses.

He didn't want to move his stuff out and locked me out of the unit. I lost out on 2 rentals of income and if you understand the short-term rental game, it can be lucrative, and I was booked for the season.

I finally convinced him to move his stuff into the RV and take the bigger items to his grandmothers. I also got him to agree to stay up at his grandmothers for a while allowing me to get the house listed and sell the RV.

Except, he didn't want to do that.

He went to his grandmothers for two days and came back, expecting to stay in the RV until the renter was gone.

He wanted to be back in the full apartment where he could come and go and not pay rent. I explained that was not an option as it was now 'in season' and I was renting it four months straight.

He was furious, he told me he was moving back up there as soon as they left and refused to let me in the RV.

I let him know the RV was going to be sold, he needed to get his stuff out, and get it cleaned. He was 29 years old and could get his own apartment!

I went to the gym, telling him his stuff needed to be out by the time I got back.

When I returned, not only was he still there, but he had broken into the main house, **MY HOUSE!**

He had filled up the truck I bought him, with my possessions. He had stolen jewelry, clothes, Dallas Cowboys memorabilia, and things he thought belonged to his father.

He went into my personal closet, in my bedroom, and just helped himself to what he wanted. He had no care for me, or the fact that I bought and paid for everything in there.

After everything I did for him, this is what I got in return. I was furious!

I demanded he open the truck and return my belongings. He refused. I pointed out he was parked in my driveway, using a truck I paid for, filled with clothes and items I owned, and he thought he could claim them.

He threatened to call the police on me if I didn't leave him alone. I pointed out, "With the phone I paid for and bought?"

I insisted he return my things and leave the property. He still refused.

I had to call the police myself and have an officer explain to him that he couldn't take my property from my house. That it was illegal for him to break in, even if he thought he had a claim because it was his father's house.

He said he just wanted his share of everything. The officer asked if his name was on the note, loan, or deed. It wasn't.

Same with the vehicles and the RV. It was all my property in my name and paid for by me, except the pickup truck that I had given to him.

The officer said he wasn't entitled to anything, which made him irate. He truly believed he was owed half of everything once I sold the house.

I gave him the pickup truck so that he could get around and I had planned on giving him some cash to get an apartment, but after this nonsense I was done.

I got my items back, and he was sent to stay with his grandmother until he could get a job and start paying rent.

But he pocketed my Jeep key and held it hostage, refusing to return it unless I gave him all his dad's property, which was legally mine. I had bought it after all.

I reached out to Tim's mom and brothers for help getting my key back, but no one seemed willing to assist. They didn't see what the big deal was.

Instead, they demanded Tim's belongings - his drum set I bought from the band Dope. My Dodge Hellcat, and one brother offered to wash it and "take it off my hands." Along with assorted Dallas Cowboys memorabilia, Tims expensive jewelry, and more.

I couldn't believe how death tears families apart and brings out the worst in people.

By the time I drove up twice to drop off Tim's items to them and try to get my Jeep key, they had ripped apart his drum set from the band Dope and kept other stuff he had stored there.

I was able to salvage what was left of the bass drum and send that along with his watch, shoes, and belt (the 3 things he loved the most) to his son Jackson in California. I wanted to split everything between the two boys so they could remember Tim in their own way.

I couldn't live in that house any longer.

It was a beautiful property but way too much for one person. I put it up for sale along with the RV and Ford pickup and walked away. I had to get back to focusing on myself and helping clients that truly want to get sober.

Looking forward to what this next chapter holds for me.

Suggested Listen:
Van Nuys by Sixx:A.M.

Acknowledgements

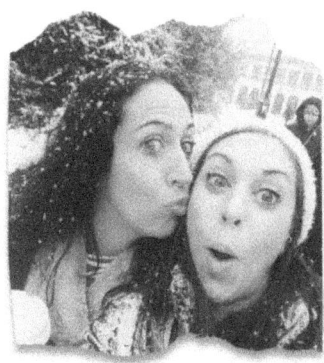

Thank you to my sister Jenny Fontana for helping me get through the living hell I was in and for being such a great ear after Tim's passing.

Thank you to Dr. Teralyn Sell for dropping everything to help me navigate widowhood and 'all the things' that need to be done.

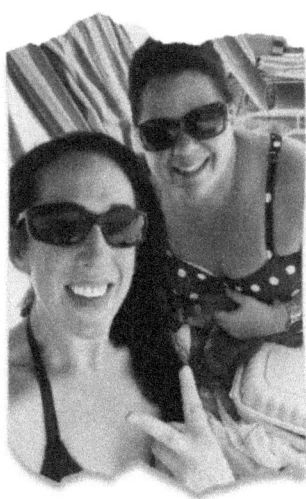

Epilogue

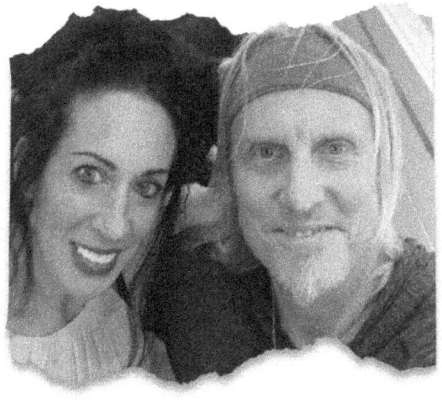

You probably think I should have left Tim in 2019 when I wanted a divorce. I tried. He refused to sign the papers. He wanted half of everything, plus alimony, and if I had agreed to that, he would have died of an overdose in less than 60 days.

I contacted an attorney and even tried to put a trust fund together that he could draw from once he got sober, but in Florida that is not an option for a spouse.

The law states that since I created my company while married, he is legally entitled to half of everything and we would have to liquidate it all, or I would have to 'buy his half' out.

Not only would I have to deal with an active drug user, but I would also need to pay him a lump sum of my company for a divorce. That lump sum would have killed him faster than his drug use complications.

It is horrific watching a spouse spiral out of control so many times and dig themselves out of the hole, only to be lured back into it.

The worst part was I knew him sober for years and he was my person. When he was sober, he was the most amazing human on the planet.

He was kind, loving, fun and positive. He never had a negative thing to say about anything or anyone. He hated conflict and we never fought-- unless it was over his drug use or spending problem. (Remember the Hellcat? Or the Crow's Nest RV?)

If you know anything about Human Design or Life Path numbers, Tim was an 11. The most creative and successful of all.

He could literally create anything by just envisioning it. Everyone loved him. He was an amazing entertainer, and we were the perfect match.

He excelled in areas I didn't and vice versa. That kind of love is hard to find. I didn't want to give it up easily, because I had had the best six years of my life with him in the beginning.

I just wanted my Tim back.

But on January 9, 2024, I finally got him to agree to a divorce and I was giving him half. I simply couldn't take it anymore.

Every detox was the last one, every trip was a make-up trip, everything was a do-over for him and he just couldn't stay sober.

I was killing myself trying to keep him alive and I was done. I had exhausted every resource I had and stayed in the marriage longer than I wanted. I needed out.

I didn't expect him to die, he always seemed to have nine lives and to cheat death. He was administered Narcan over five times and had all those accidents. Plus, his hepatic artery burst, and he survived a major bleed that only 1 % survived.

I had received calls from hospitals, police officers, jails, and he always walked away - unscathed. This caught up to him and I wasn't ready for it.

That is why I didn't plan a Celebration of Life or publish this book sooner. I needed time to heal and process it all.

We were writing this book when he died and his chapters, he penned himself.

Sometimes I think he knew he was going to die and that is why he left that day and went to Naples. He always said, "It's been a good run." His run just ran out.

I am thankful to be able to publish this book. I want everyone to see the human side of addiction and what a spouse goes through.

There are a lot of books for parents of a child that has addiction issues, but few that a spouse can relate to.

Hopefully this book brought laughter and tears for you and if you know anyone struggling to get sober and leave drugs and alcohol behind, please reach out for help.

Dr. Cali Estes & Tim Estes

"See you on the Flip Side" ~ Cali Estes and Tim

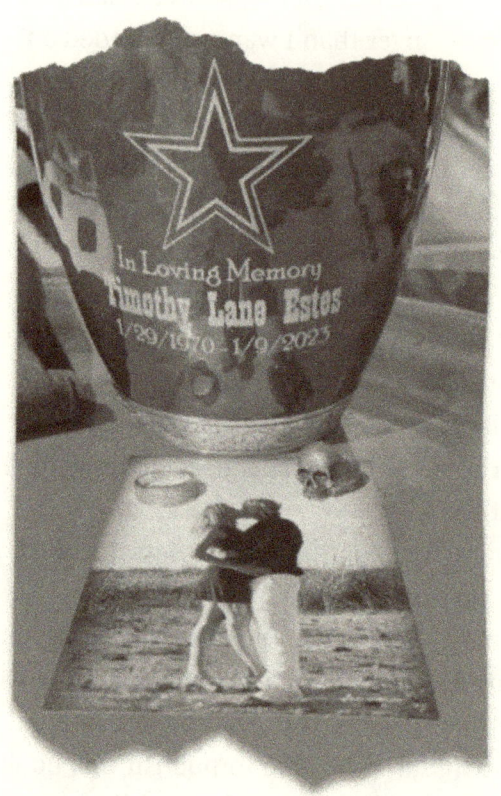

Suggested song:
Lost Soul's Prayer by Brantley Gilbert

Tales from the Road

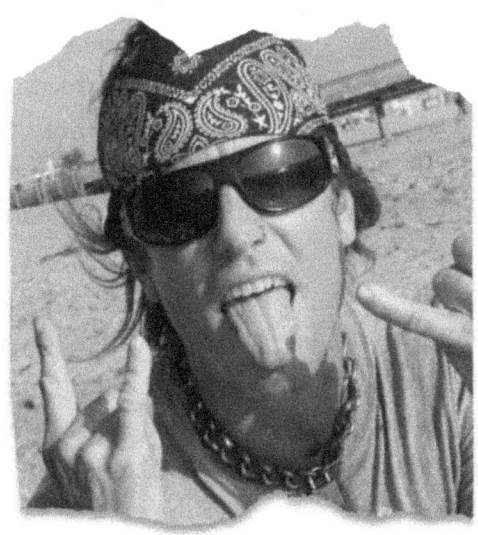

Rock 'n' roll isn't just about the music—it's about the journey, the misadventures, and the stories that become legend. In this section, we dive into the wild world of Crowfly and The Deadlyz, as recounted by Brandon James and Jon Moody, offering two unique perspectives on the unpredictable life of Tim Estes.

These tales, featuring Tim and his bandmates, offer a raw, unfiltered glimpse into the chaotic life of touring rock bands in their early days. From New York City mishaps to cross-country tours in a beat-up van, accidental border crossing fiascos to run-ins with the law, these stories capture the essence of what it means to be young, reckless, and driven by an unquenchable passion for music.

Brandon James, lead singer of Crowfly, adds another layer to Tim's story, sharing shocking accounts of Tim's struggles with addiction and the band's attempts to navigate the unpredictable nature of performing with a functioning addict. His stories highlight both the magic and the mayhem that Tim brought to their music, showcasing the complex relationship between creativity and destruction.

Prepare yourself for a rollercoaster ride of laughter, disbelief, and nostalgia as we journey through the untamed landscape of these bands' rise to infamy. These aren't just stories—they're snapshots of a lifestyle few dare to live and even fewer survive to tell about.

From near-death experiences during practice sessions to chaotic benefit concerts for bikers, these tales paint a vivid picture of Tim Estes—a man of incredible talent and passion, whose addiction often threatened to overshadow his gifts.

So strap in, turn up the volume, and get ready to hit the road with The Deadlyz and Crowfly. It's going to be one hell of a ride—unpredictable, intense, and unforgettable, just like Tim himself.

I Married A Junkie – The Final Chapter

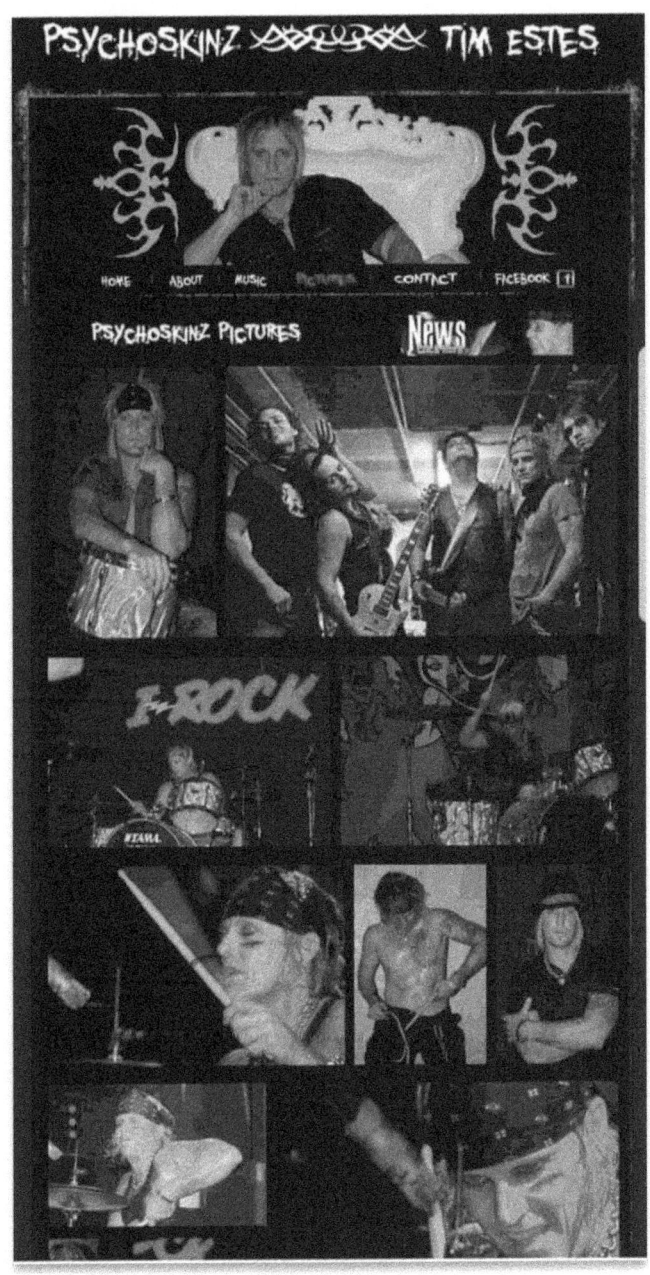

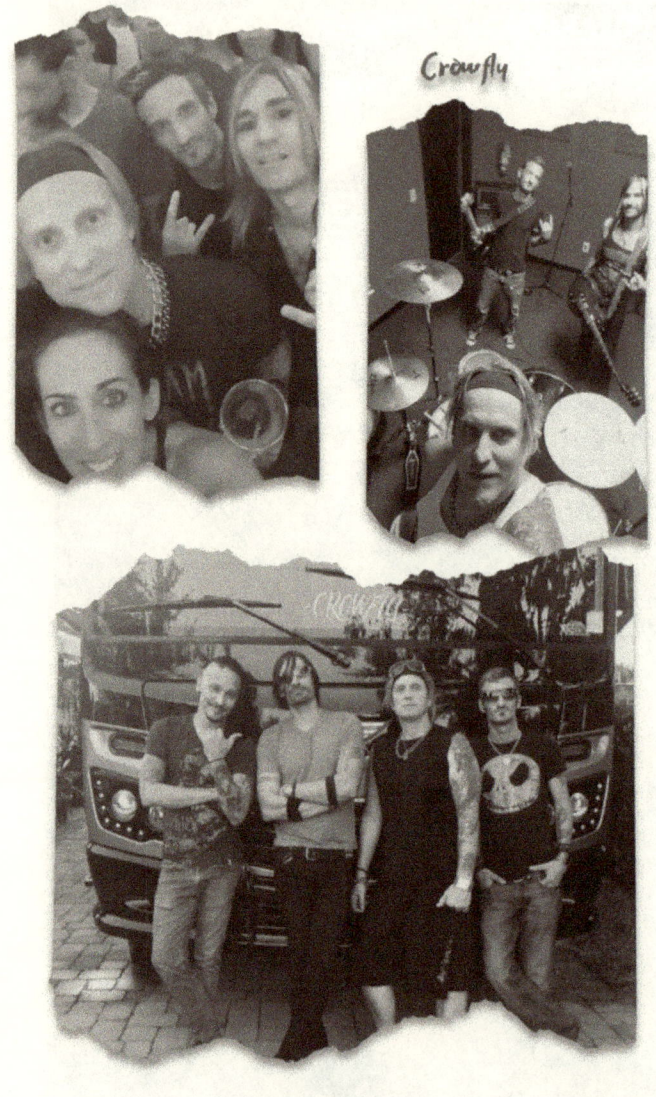

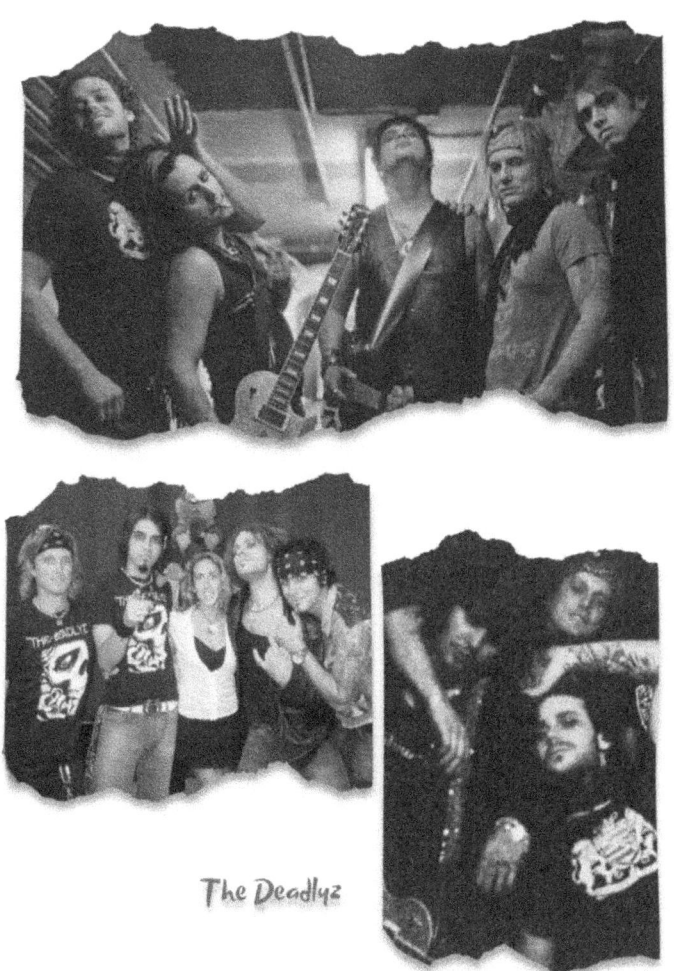

The Deadlyz

Brandon James
Lead Singer, Crowfly

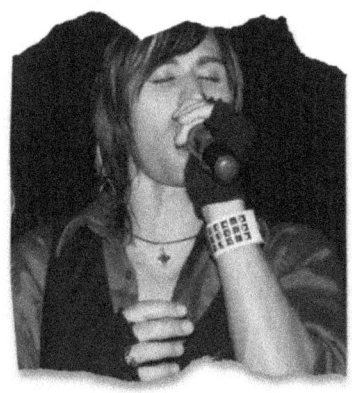

When I say Timothy was unpredictable, that is no exaggeration. In fact, it's an understatement. I have known him for a long time and as a lead singer in several projects, I got to know Tim very well.

When I think back to all the people I have met in the music industry, no one stands out more than Timothy Estes. He was a man with incredible drive, talent, and passion but was always hindered by an uncontrollable addiction.

I knew Timothy for approximately 10 years. During that time, I watched him overdose, get ridiculously high, and even die on multiple occasions. No drug was off limits, but heroin and cocaine were his favorites. Usually, one balanced out the other as he would use these together quite often.

One instance that my bandmates and I will never forget is a late-night practice where he died and came back to life, at least from our perspective. Being the drummer of our band, Tim was already exerting himself during a three-hour practice session. It was not uncommon for him to do a few lines of coke before practice, and on this night, we didn't think much of it when we saw him pour a few lines on his snare drum.

We practiced for about two hours and took a small break. Before we started up again, our Argentinian bass player Lucia, usually the voice of reason in the band, noticed a bag of heroin on Tim's snare drum.

While giving Tim a worried frown, he said, "I don't think that's a good idea."

Of course, Tim completely ignored the warning and proceeded to snort half the bag of heroin. He did this off the top of his snare drum while he was playing. We all could not believe our eyes and were in even more disbelief of how accurately he kept the beat while pulling this off.

We kept playing and finished the song. Shortly after, Tim leaned back against the wall and said, "We need a break."

We could tell he was not feeling well and looked higher than the star Polaris. We agreed to take a break, and Tim stayed back while we stepped outside for some air.

When we returned, we found Tim completely laid out on the floor. He was not breathing. Not at all. We knew he might be gone and didn't have time to call paramedics.

We picked him up and tried to sit him upright. When we did this, he made a small grunt and then a cough. He was barely alive from what we could tell. Lucia probably saved his life by suggesting we give him more cocaine. The mix of heroin and coke is why he was in this mess, to begin with, but it sounded like a reasonable idea at the time.

We poured a small amount on the tip of his tongue and gave him a healthy smack across the face. Maybe this restarted his heart.

Tim's eyes opened, and he started coughing again. We were all scared stiff until he finally broke a smile and said,

"What's up, guys?" He was obviously clueless as to what had just happened.

A few minutes later, he was back on his feet and ready to get back to practice. Of course, we all declined and called it a night, not knowing what the hell had just happened.

It was times like these that made every minute with Tim completely unpredictable.

~

Being in a band with a junkie kept things interesting. Never once was there a dull moment, especially while touring. Some days I wonder how we were able to put on a professional rock show with all the chaos that ensued just before we hit the stage.

Once, we did a benefit concert for kids with disabilities. It was hosted by a very large group of bikers.

The show was not designed for bands, there was no real stage or sound setup. It was more just for bands and fans to get together to have fun and for a good cause.

When it was our turn, we took the stage, which was basically a circus tent over a slab of concrete. Tim was already high well before we took the stage.

During our setup and soundcheck, I mentioned I was feeling a little tired. He said he had some energy drinks and would give me a small amount in a cup just to give me a boost.

Now, after knowing Tim for several years by this point, I should have known better, but I was tired and didn't think much of it. Well, what he gave me was a triple dose of C4, which is basically pure caffeine and designed to work very rapidly.

I had such an adverse reaction to it that I could barely speak, much less sing. It also made me itch uncontrollably, and it was downright miserable. I did not find the humor in this whatsoever.

Because I couldn't sing, I knew we were going to sound like shit, and the rest of the band didn't even want to play at all. Well, to make matters worse, we had a 30-minute set. Tim decided about five minutes in that he was not going to continue. He didn't like the setup situation, and he said he couldn't hear.

I can't say I didn't agree with him, but we had a job to do, and I felt we should finish the set. Well, we did not finish. Tim walked off stage, leaving the rest of us feeling like idiots.

Now, I don't know a whole lot about bikers, but I found out that day they were not very forgiving. They were extremely pissed and basically wanted to beat the hell out of our drummer.

They searched for him for quite some time before giving up. Afraid they might take it out on us, we packed up our stuff faster than we ever did before and left the scene before it got ugly.

Things like this would make most bands break up and move on. But we loved Tim. Everyone did. And the chemistry we had and the magic that happened in that band was just worth it. It was worth all the chaos and the destruction. I never met a functioning heroin addict like Timothy.

One thing I still hear over and over in my head is our bassist Lucia saying, "Tim is destroyed."

We all got used to him saying that. And we would all just answer, "Yes, we know."

Tim could just keep going, and because of this, we just kept doing what we were doing. Looking back, we all should have played a bigger part in trying to get him sober. I am not sure if we could have, though. I'm not sure anyone could.

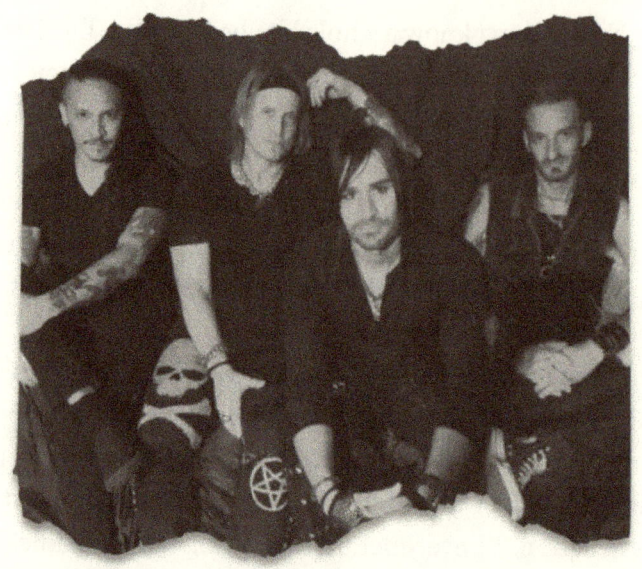

Suggested Listen: <u>Lit Up by Buckcherry</u>

Jon Moody
Lead Singer, The Deadlyz

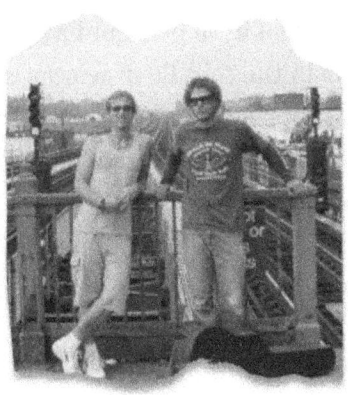

When we first got to New York and started this band, we lived in this musician building on 51st and 8th. It was awesome, just two blocks away from Times Square. It was easy access to work and all the trouble we could conjure up.

One day we decided to go down to Lower Manhattan. We had Metro cards that you could use for a 24-hour period, so we figured we could hop on and off all over town. What we didn't realize was that the MetroCard could only be used one time there and one time back. We came up with this fabulous plan: Tim was going to go through, then I was going to jump the turnstile.

Great idea, Tim, except we didn't realize there were a couple of cops on the other side waiting for people just like us. The train just happened to pull up, and when the doors opened, we scrambled in. The doors closed just in time, and we evaded getting a ticket or possible arrest.

We figured we'd go down to the Staten Island Ferry, hang out by the river a little bit, and have some fun. Keep in mind, this was in the middle of winter, and none of us were dressed appropriately: eyeliner, skinny rock 'n' roll jeans, and the smallest jacket you could wear to keep the rock 'n' roll look.

I remember Tim saying, "Hey, hold onto this MetroCard for me because I don't have any pockets." He was wearing new rock 'n' roll wear he'd purchased in Saint Marks a couple of days prior. I put the MetroCard into my back pocket, which, of course, had a hole in it.

A couple of hours later, after our drunk walk around and sightseeing, Tim said, "Let's go back to Hell's Kitchen." I went to grab the MetroCard, but it had fallen out of my pocket. We had no way to get back to where we lived on 51st and 8th, so we had to walk all the way from the Staten Island Ferry. Keep in mind, we only had one pint of vodka to share between the both of us - that just wasn't enough.

I remember there was a liquor store on the corner of about 34th Street. Manhattan wasn't as locked down then, so you could walk in and see the product on the shelf. Tim used me as a distraction to ask about different bottles of wine. I kept the clerk busy while Tim swiped a bottle, sticking it in his jacket and walking out. When I figured that was enough time, I said, "Okay, maybe tomorrow we'll just get another bottle of Merlot," wrote down the bottle on a piece of paper, thanked the clerk, and walked out.

The next day, Tim and I decided to go to Central Park to work on some ideas for the song "Retox." We grabbed ourselves a bottle of vodka and went to Central Park. I had my old computer from 2005 - no Wi-Fi capability, real technology. We set up the computer and started working on some music, set up the microphone and stand, and I was recording vocals to some of the pre-recorded ideas we had on the computer.

Our music is loud rock 'n' roll party music, so of course, there's some yelling and screaming. The cops in the area heard the commotion and wanted to see what was going on. They came out of nowhere in unmarked vehicles and civilian clothing, catching us with open containers and a bottle of vodka.

We all got citations and needed to go downtown Brooklyn to pay this fine. It doesn't end there - we decided on our day off to go pay the bill at the courthouse in Brooklyn. We thought it'd be a fantastic idea to pre-game with vodka and cranberry juice before we went in to pay the bill. We smelled like a couple of homeless bums going in there and almost got arrested for public intoxication.

~

I remember when we did our first road tour with the band, we first had to find a roadworthy vehicle. A bus wasn't in our budget, but we found a 1984 Econoline van, the type that Mr. T would have driven. Once we secured this van, we all took a trip down to Florida to purchase this new addition to the band.

We were only about an hour and a half on the road when the van started doing a jump and wobble, and then POW! Yep, that was the tire. We changed the blown-out tire with the spare under the vehicle and continued our trip. Exactly half an hour later, the second tire blew. We pulled off and magically found a replacement at a Chevron gas station and continued our journey.

I kid you not, not even an hour and a half later, 70 miles down the road, tires number three and four blew out at exactly the same time. So we were stuck on the side of the highway right next to a Walmart with no money and no food. We decided to go to Walmart and see what the cheapest thing was we could fill our bodies with. You guessed it - beer is what we wish we could've had, but because it was Sunday, they had restrictions on buying alcohol. So, our next best thing, of course, was NyQuil - 10% alcohol. We decided to get obliterated on cough medicine.

Fast-forward to another trip with the same vehicle. We were driving to our very first show in Albuquerque, New Mexico. It was supposed to be a packed show - all tickets were sold, and we were headlining. We were driving in that old beat-up 1980s Econoline van through Texas, and about three-quarters of the way, our lights went out. No headlights.

We pulled over and devised a fantastic plan to stick a flashlight in one of the windows so we could have lights to see on the freeway. Of course, you can imagine that the state troopers weren't excited about that idea. We ended up getting pulled over and interrogated. We had all our band stuff on - chains, spikes, makeup, the whole nine yards - and of course, an open case of beer and an illegal bass player with no papers.

Right before the van came to a stop, we all looked at Gabriel and said, "Okay, you've got an accent, buddy. It's time to learn how to speak Southern, and you're from Missouri, alright?" He got the accent down pretty good, but when the cop asked where we were from and Gabriel responded he was from Missouri, it opened up a can of worms. That state trooper just happened to be from Missouri.

Tim distracted him by offering to show him our flyer. The cop looked at it and said, "Sex, drugs, rock 'n' roll, and mayhem," then asked if there were drugs in the van. We explained it was just a rock 'n' roll persona to make the music look tougher.

The cop said we wouldn't make it to Albuquerque that night and made us pull off at a motel. He told us, "You're gonna stay the night. During the day you're free to drive because you don't need headlights." We waited until the cop was gone, then decided to continue our journey into Albuquerque, New Mexico, with absolutely no headlights and a flashlight for our guide.

~

Here's a story I'll absolutely never forget from when we were on that little tour with that same messed up van. I say messed up - it barely had any seats. The flooring was gone right down to the bare metal, but it still carried our asses all the way from New York City to Los Angeles, California.

We had a show to play at the Whisky a Go Go out there in LA. The bass player didn't have an amp; he just came with his bass, so he needed to borrow a bass amp for the show. No problem. Tim knew some people out there in LA from one of his previous bands, so we just borrowed an amp from one of those guys.

We played the show, but when we finished, security came up and took the bass player's bass away. The bass player looked at us, looked at Tim, looked at the security, and said, "What are you doing?" The security guy said, "Well, you were supposed to sell a certain number of tickets, and you didn't sell tickets, so we gotta use something as collateral."

Long story short, Tim worked out a deal where they would hold the bass as collateral until we could get the money to the Whisky a Go Go, and then we'd get the bass back once it was paid off. No problem, we left. Gabriel had to leave his bass there, but we still had the bass amp we borrowed. This amp was borrowed from Tim's friend, who had borrowed it from some mafia mobsters, and we had a deadline to get that bass amp back.

We forgot that we had the bass amp and forgot to give it back, so we were being hunted all over LA. We couldn't give it back to the original owner it was borrowed from. Absolutely crazy and true story.

On that little tour we took, there's one story that has got to be told and heard. We were on our way back from doing a show in Chicago and going up to visit my parents with the band so we could get some relaxed time in.

Everybody knows that when driving through Detroit, there is an exit that goes into Windsor, Canada. This exit is very tricky because it says, "Follow the sign to Detroit," but if you're not paying attention to this little, tiny 12x12 sign that says "Downtown," you would immediately go right into Border Patrol, which there is absolutely no exit from.

So, you have to go into customs to get passport and vehicle checks. Well, none of us had passports, one of us had multiple felonies, and the bass player was illegal from Brazil. Once the Canadian customs found out our situation - oh, and don't forget there were empty beer cans and open bottles everywhere in that van - they had an absolute field day with us.

They had the bass player in the back room detained, Tim talking to one of the border patrol officers, and me and the guitar player in a whole other section. Long story short, they gave us these pieces of paper which they taped onto the windshield, two of them to be exact. One was for the deportation of the bass player once we got over to the

US territory side, to immediately take him into custody to be deported back to Brazil. And another note stating that we could never come back into Canada ever again.

We had to devise a plan very quickly because that would end our band immediately. Before we got up to the entry zone back into the US, we decided to take the piece of paper that said to deport the bass player back to Brazil, wadded it up, and threw it in the back of the van. So, all they saw was "Don't let them back into Canada ever again."

I don't know how we got out of that crazy situation, but we managed to get out with our bass player and everybody on US soil. I think Tim kept that Canadian piece of paper and stuck it on our apartment wall in Manhattan. He was proud of that.

I Married A Junkie – The Final Chapter

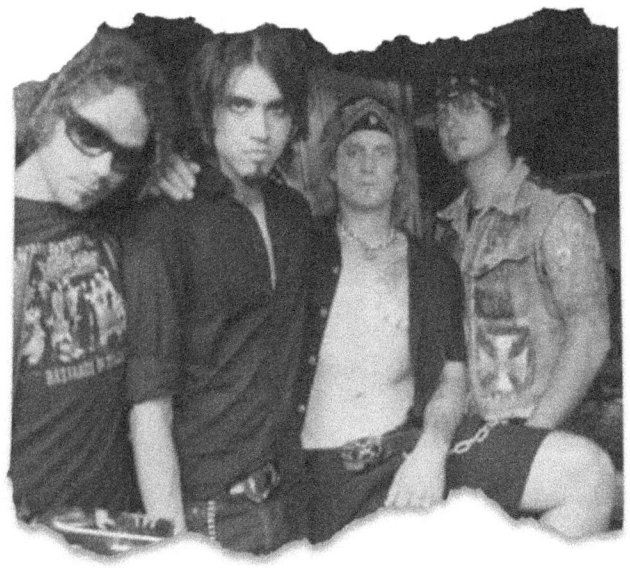

Suggested Listen: <u>Unraveling by Sevendust</u>

Thank You

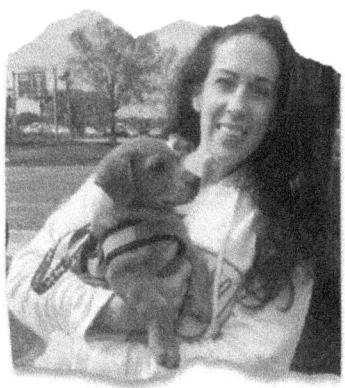

Dr. Cali Estes continues to focus her work on helping others with her multiple pathways to recovery from addiction and mental health.

You can learn more about Dr. Estes and her work at:
www.IMarriedAJunkie.com (Best Selling Books)
www.SoberOnDemand.com (for clients)
www.TheAddictionCoachOnline.com (for clients)
www.CaliEstes.com
www.TheAddictionsAcademy.com (for students)
www.AAMHT.com (for students)
www.UnpauseYourLife.com
www.ProRecoveryRX.com (supplements)

Thank you again for your support and you can get access to color photographs and more that were not included in the book at: www.IMarriedAJunkie.com

www.ingramcontent.com/pod-product-compliance
Lightning Source LLC
Chambersburg PA
CBHW032118090426
42743CB00007B/385